Training Handbook of Mental Disorders in Individuals with Intellectual Disability

Edited by

Nancy N. Cain, M.D.
Geraldine Holt, M.B.B.S., B.Sc., F.R.C. Psych.
Phillip W. Davidson, Ph.D.
Nick Bouras, M.D, Ph.D., F.R.C. Psych.

Copyright © 2006 NADD Press

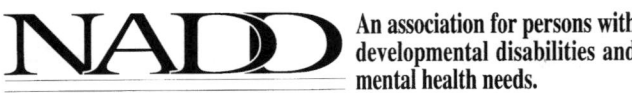 An association for persons with developmental disabilities and mental health needs.

132 Fair Street
Kingston, New York 12401

All rights reserved.

No part of this book may be reproduced, stored in a retrieval system or transmitted in any form by means of electronic, mechanical, photocopy, recording or otherwise, without written permission of NADD, 132 Fair Street, Kingston, New York, 12401

LCCN: 2006922813
ISBN: 1-57256-021-5

1st Printing 2006

Printed in the United States of America

Table of Contents

Overview
Philip W. Davidson, Nancy N. Cain 1

Assessment of Mental Disorders in Individuals with Intellectual Disability
John C. Pomeroy 15

Mental Disorders in Adults with Intellectual Disability
Howard B. Demb 33

Presentation of Mental Disorders in Children and Adolescents with Intellectual Disability
Howard B. Demb 55

Prevalence of Behavioral Disturbance
John W. Jacobson 87

Autism
Caroline I. Magyar, Tristram Smith, Jennifer Katz 99

Psychotherapeutic Interventions
Joanne T. Baxter, Nancy N. Cain 115

Applied Behavioral Analysis
Peter Sturmey, Howie Reyer, Ronald Lee, Adrienne Robek 131

Psychotropic Medications
Nancy N. Cain, Anthony Villani 147

Community-Based Mental Health Services
Nick Bouras, Geraldine Holt, Amy Cowley 165

Ethical and Legal Issues
Christine D. Cea, Celia B. Fisher 177

Acknowledgements

We are indebted to those leaders in the field who went before us, who shared their knowledge and enthusiasm to carry this work forward. We appreciate our colleagues who have supported us in our clinical work and in the development of our understanding of the presentation of mental disorders in individuals with ID. We thank our clients and their caregivers, who have taught us a great deal, and with whom we are still learning. We are grateful to Cathy Imhof and Christina McCrone for their expert assistance in the final preparations of the manuscript. The senior editor, Nancy Cain, also wishes to thank her husband, Russell M. Cain, M.D., for the wisdom and support he has provided.

Preface

This book is intended to be used as a basic introduction for any service provider beginning to work with individuals who have the dual diagnoses of both mental retardation (MR), herein identified as intellectual disability (ID), and mental illness or psychiatric disorders, hereafter identified as mental disorders. As more and more institutions close, individuals with both ID and a mental disorder, those generally most difficult to care for, now live within the general community. Thus, clinicians and care providers throughout the United States are being asked to care for individuals with very complex problems—problems that require an interdisciplinary team using a biopsychosocial model for accurate assessment, diagnosis, treatment, and care. Without an understanding of these individuals and the available tools to serve them, clinicians and caregivers find themselves at a loss to help, which can lead to turning the client away. Many clinicians and caregivers, however, want to learn how to work with individuals with both ID and a mental disorder. It is our intention to provide, both those new to the field and those still learning, with basic information to guide them and strengthen their skills so that they may best serve this population with such complex problems.

This book grew out of the awareness that there were too few care providers who understood and were therefore comfortable with people who had both ID and a mental disorder, but many of them wanted to acquire a better understanding. Many colleagues told us that it would be very helpful to them if we wrote a book to share what we had learned over our years of providing psychiatric care to individuals with both ID and a mental disorder. The opportunity arose to act on this request when the four editors began considering how to best modify a training manual that Dr. Geraldine Holt and Professor Nick Bouras had published in the United Kingdom, so that it would be applicable for use in the United States.

We hope that this book will also provide basic information about intellectual disability and mental disorders for graduate school courses. The needs of individuals with ID and mental disorders should be brought to the attention of students early in their training, as most all of them will encounter them in whatever type of human service they choose. This will be true, for example, for medical students who become internists or surgeons, speech pathologists that enter a clinic practice, or social workers that work in general hospitals. Plus, such students might make the choice to specialize in work with individuals with both ID and a mental disorder, if they are aware of the field. We hope that this book will stimulate interest in working with individuals who have both ID and a mental disorder and inspire some to become experts and leaders in the field.

The work is quite challenging as it involves dealing with two disorders, each of which can cause cognitive and affective impairments and socially inappropriate behaviors. However, it can be quite rewarding to have the appropriate tools to best determine what is happening and how to intervene to improve a person's quality of life. We also hope that this book will be one of those tools so that more and more individuals with ID and a mental disorder receive the quality care that they need.

We have organized this book into two sections: the disorders and the treatments. The first chapter describes the field and sets the work in a historical context. Since a good assessment is essential to determine the type of needed care, this follows in Chapter Two. The next four chapters identify many of the mental disorders seen in individuals with ID and gives examples of how to identify such signs and symptoms. The second half of the book focuses on a variety of treatments and then looks at one example of a comprehensive community system for providing care. It concludes with a discussion and guidance on some of the legal and ethical issues that need to be kept in mind.

Over the years, as treatment has become more person-centered, clinicians and consumers have found many of the terms used to describe the individual with a disability as pejorative and dehumanizing. Labels are used to categorize or to define the contents or characteristics of something. Finding the best description that identifies the disability without demeaning the person can be difficult, in part, because there are many different opinions. Many organizations and providers have been grappling with this, and much of the terminology is still in flux. In responding to this, several international organizations have changed from using MR to using ID. Most countries other than the U.S. also use ID. Though mental retardation remains the term used in the U.S., President Bush recently renamed The President's Committee on MR to The President's Committee on ID.

For clarity throughout this book, we have made editorial decisions regarding usage of terms. We apologize to anyone who is uncomfortable with our choices and hope that this will not detract from the book's message: individuals, whether called people with MR or ID, who also have a mental disorder(s), need specialized care and treatment.

Individuals with ID span a wide range of abilities and many feel demeaned when called retarded. In an era when people with disabilities have fought for equal rights, the opportunities to live life with dignity and have person-centered planning to meet their needs, it is important to view a person as someone with a disability in a specific area, not as a dysfunctional subject. The term "mental retardation" has too often carried with it the pejorative view that people with ID are unable to do anything but remain like young children who need total care and supervision.

Likewise, mental illness and psychiatric disorders or illnesses are loaded terms for most people in the American culture. Many university outpatient programs have dropped the word "psychiatric" from the names of their facilities and instead call themselves Behavioral Health Centers. This is unfortunate because it essentially removes the psyche from focus and does not emphasize subjective psychological or emotional components of diagnosis, treatment, and care. However to the layperson, mental illness or the need for psychiatric care may carry a stigma, and most individuals do not want to be labeled as such. "Illness" is less acceptable language, as it draws on the traditional medical model and some of the paternalistic approaches that have been a part of it. To minimize this dilemma we have chosen to use the term "mental disorders," as used in both the Diagnostic and Statistical Manual of Mental Disorders (DSM-IV-TR) of the American Psychiatric Association and the World Health Organization's International Classification of Diseases (ICD-10). Therefore, throughout this book the term "mental disorders" will be used whereever the terms "mental illness" or "psychiatric disorder" may have traditionally been used.

We avoided using: "patient" for which we use "client," "consumer," or "individual." We have also chosen not to use "behavior disorders," because these are not yet well defined. Instead we use "behavior disturbance," since we believe that most of these disturbances are caused or maintained by a mental disorder or an environmental factor.

We hope that you will find this book helpful and wish you well in your work in this challenging and rewarding field, and that some of you will go on to continue the development of the much-needed services for individuals with ID and mental disorders.

Foreword
Ludwik S. Szymanski

Not many today are aware that the humane approaches to care for persons with Intellectual Disabilities were originally initiated by psychiatrists. In the United States, physicians such as Edouard Sequin and Samuel Gridley pioneered the enlightened care based on educational principles, with optimistic goals of habilitation and return to the community as its productive members. All founders of the precursor of the American Association on Intellectual Disabilities in 1876 were medical directors of residential facilities for persons with Intellectual Disabilities. Yet, over the years and until recently, psychiatry (and other mental health professions) had not followed these pioneers, and Intellectual Disabilities remained a sort of "Cinderella" of organized psychiatry and psychology. However, an increasing number of professionals, such as Drs. Harry Potter, George Tarjan, and Frank Menolascino dedicated themselves to research, clinical services, and training professionals in the field of psychiatry of Intellectual Disabilities. It is my guess that they influenced many of the contributors to this book (as well as myself).

In the 1960s, the normalization movement emerged from Scandinavia, and it was followed by de-institutionalization of persons with Intellectual Disabilities. The number of persons living in large, state institutions declined from the peak of 194,650 in 1967 to 52, 801 in 1998 (Braddock, 2000). On the other hand, the number of persons residing in the community increased. Great strides have been made in preparing individuals with Intellectual Disabilities for achieving good quality of life, through appropriate education, vocational training, and provision of support services. At the same time it became obvious that disturbed behavior, usually a result of an underlying and often undiagnosed mental disorder, was the prime obstacle to successful community integration of persons with Intellectual Disabilities. Many research studies in several countries (reviewed in this book) documented the high vulnerability of these individuals to mental and behavioral disorders, due to combined effects of high prevalence of neuropathology and high level of environmental stresses coupled with low coping skills. In many cases a behavioral phenotype may be discerned: the Intellectual Disability is associated with a genetic syndrome, in which psychiatric symptomatology is a part of the clinical presentation. All this has led to a dramatic increase in the need for mental health services for this population.

As the result of legislation, court decisions and their own empowerment, persons with Intellectual Disabilities are entitled now to receive medical care including mental health care and may be even more eligible than many in the general population, since an overwhelming majority are insured under Medicaid or Medicare. However, lack of trained mental health professionals, psychiatrists, in particular, has been the major obstacle to their access to mental health care. Relatively few graduate-training programs provide training in developmental disabilities to residents in psychiatry (American Psychiatric Association, 1998). Mental health professionals untrained in this field have difficulty in diagnosing mental disorders in persons with limited language skills and tend to resort to a narrow range of treatment approaches. While these may be sufficient in typical psychiatric clients with mental disorders, who need to return to their premorbid state, persons with Intellectual Disabilities need a comprehensive treatment and habilitation program based on biopsychosocial approaches. Lately, the situation has been made worse by pressure from health insurers for quick symptomatic treatment, usually with medications only. Thus, the need for trained providers of primary mental health care in medical and non-medical disciplines is acute and growing.

This book is an important step in the right direction toward satisfying this need. The existing training materials such as textbooks and book chapters on psychiatry of Intellectual Disabilities are usually oriented toward training sub-specialists. This book is unique in that it provides a broad overview of the field as well as practical information concerning diagnostic, treatment, and support techniques that are useful for professionals in a broad range of disciplines and training levels. It promotes an interdisciplinary approach based on a biopsychosocial orientation, to diagnosis and treatment. Respect for individual rights and autonomy is highlighted and even a separate chapter is devoted to this topic. It should become an important training aid and resource for diverse groups of professionals, including psychiatrists, psychologists, social workers, nurses, and primary care physicians who care for persons with Intellectual Disabilities, as well as for direct care providers.

REFERENCES
American Psychiatric Association, 1998

1

Overview

Philip W. Davidson and Nancy N. Cain

INTRODUCTION

To advocate for and work with individuals with mental retardation, referred heretofore as Intellectual Disabilities (ID), and mental disorders most effectively, it is important to have an historical perspective of each classification. It is also important to understand the terminology used in both the mental health and the ID service systems as they differ significantly. This chapter outlines the historical, political and social forces that have influenced care over the past two centuries. Though the book focuses on ID, this chapter begins with a discussion of developmental disabilities (DD), as ID is one of the clusters of DD. After reading this chapter, readers should not only be able to define DD and ID but also have an understanding of the historical events leading to the current status of services and supports for people with ID who also have a mental disorder(s) or behavioral disturbance(s). They should also have an understanding of the evolution of care models from medieval times to the present day as well as be able to describe some of the settings within which care was provided and explain the eventual split of the two provider systems. Many stresses impact the individual, family and caregivers that can lead to a worsening of underlying mental disorders. Individuals with ID and a mental disorder(s) can experience entry into care systems particularly difficult. This book intends to give the reader some real understanding of this challenge.

OVERVIEW OF DEVELOPMENTAL DISABILITIES

DD includes several diagnostic groupings or disorders that collectively affect between 2% and 3% of the U.S. population (Levy, 1996). The most prevalent of these disorders is ID, thought to occur in about 1% of the U.S. population (Batshaw & Shapiro, 2002). Other DDs include neuromotor disorders such as cerebral palsy, autism spectrum disorders and neurological disorders, for example, childhood-onset epilepsy and Tourette's disorder. There are several common elements that tie these diverse diagnoses together. Based upon the U.S. Government's definition, they are all severe, chronic impairments. They all originate and exert their effects during the developmental period, that is, before age 22 years, and cause life-long impairments in functions such as cognition, language, motor abilities, perception, learning and adaptive behavior. They all may interfere with an individual's economic and social self-sufficiency and impair their ability to lead independent lives as fully integrated members of society.

CLINICAL DEFINITIONS OF DEVELOPMENTAL DISABILITIES

Until the 1970s, individuals with disabilities were grouped according to predominant medical diagnosis. Each group had separate organizations for evaluation, treatment, ongoing care and political lobbying. Individuals with ID were classified according to diagnostic criteria determined by professional organizations such as the American Association on Mental Retardation or the American Academy of Cerebral Palsy. Other specific disabilities were defined by international classification systems such as the Diagnostic and Statistical Manual of Mental Disorders (DSM-IV-TR) of the American Psychiatric Association (2000) and the World Health Organization's International Classification of Diseases (ICD-10) (1992). In each case, the disability was diagnosed according to physical or medical characteristics. For example, ID was classified by its effect on intellectual ability and adaptive behavior (AAMR, 2002), and cerebral palsy was classified on the basis of the type, severity and scope of the neuromotor impairment (Black, 1999). This clinical approach has several benefits:

- It yields a clear picture of the clinical impact of each disorder;
- It affords clinicians with a metric to gauge the design and success of treatments and interventions;
- It tends to isolate DD from mental disorders that may not appear until later in life, or that may not have their primary impact on intellectual or physical development, and
- It lends itself readily to classification of disease, a characteristic highly valued by the medical community and by government regulators and policy-makers.

However, clinical diagnostic approaches do not easily permit the estimation of the impact of the disability upon functionality: the consequences of the disability in terms of daily life functions and behaviors, the abilities that determine the degree to which an individual can function in society and the degree and type of support that they will need to increase their functional abilities.

FUNCTIONAL DEFINITIONS OF DEVELOPMENTAL DISABILITIES

In the early 1970s clinicians, policy-makers, family members and persons with disabilities began to see the benefits of combining these disabilities into a single grouping (Scheerenberger, 1987).

In 1978, the U.S. Congress amended legislation governing the rights of individuals with disabilities, now called the Developmental Disabilities Bill of Rights and Assistance Act, to include a functional definition of DD. The definition stated that a developmental disability was a severe, chronic disability attributable to a physical or mental impairment that occurred before age 22 years; that caused substantial functional limitations in three or more daily life functions, including self-care, receptive and expressive language, learning, mobility, self-direction, capacity for independent living and economic self-sufficiency, and that required individualized life-long intervention (PL-95-602; Crocker, 1987). This definition has several important features and impacts:

- It ties the disparate individual disabilities together by describing the similar impact that they have on functional ability;

- It provides the beginning of an operational definition of the consequences of the disability, introducing the potential for better treatments and measurements of treatment impact;
- It also creates the potentially negative consequence of reducing the number of persons impaired by the disorders, even though they may actually still have the clinical diagnosis of that disorder. For example, the functional ability in some people with very mild clinical symptoms may not be sufficiently affected to qualify them as individuals with DD. This consequence, in effect, compromises access to services and supports, leading to an otherwise preventable loss of functional ability at some future time, and
- It may blur the distinction between DD and mental disorders that begin and manifest during infancy and childhood. Coincident DD and mental disorders may be an example of this consequence. Often, it is difficult to distinguish which of the two conditions is etiologically primary.

This publication uses both clinical and functional definitions. Attempts by some professional organizations to strengthen the functional diagnostic approach by focusing on supports and services needed by an affected individual and their families have been met with opposition by many clinicians (Jacobson & Mulick, 1995). On the other hand, the focus on functionality has proven very useful in stimulating the development of new approaches to measuring the impact of disabilities on life functions and quality of life. There is clearly value to both approaches.

TERMINOLOGY

The dialogue concerning clinical and functional approaches to defining DD is indirectly associated with an important focus on the use of terminology to describe affected individuals. There has been growing worldwide concern about the adverse human rights effects of labeling individuals who have disabilities with diagnostic terms that may be perceived by them or by society as pejorative. Some countries have adopted the recommendations of individuals with disabilities and their advocates to change these terms to make them less pejorative and more descriptive. For example, the U.K. uses the term "learning disability" to describe persons who have ID. In many parts of Europe and Asia, the term "intellectual disability" has already replaced "mental retardation". In the early 1990s the largest international professional scientific organization addressing DD dropped the term Mental Retardation from its name, changing its designation to the International Association for the Scientific Study of Intellectual Disabilities. In 2002, the Board of Directors of the American Association on Mental Retardation recommended to its membership a change in its name to the American Association on Intellectual Disabilities. The proposal was defeated but the issue continues to be debated.

LIFE STRESSORS

Early Life Issues

The life course of an individual with DD can have a major impact on his or her well-being and mental health as well as that of the family and other caregivers. Some DD can be identified during the prenatal period, such as Down syndrome (Batshaw, 2002). It is more likely that identification may not occur until after birth or even later. The process often begins with questions about the child's development, raised either by the family or by the primary care pediatrician. These discussions typically lead to screening and ultimately to some type of evaluation to diagnose the child's disability and to prepare a plan for intervention. These events may take time and sometimes are not immediately definitive. The complexities of some DD, coupled with the lack of ability to predict the future, may prevent a definitive diagnosis or the identification of effective treatments. This is especially true in the case of children and adults with ID and mental disorders. The uncertainties of diagnosis and treatment efficacy introduce chronic stressors to the family and ultimately may have an adverse effect on the client's development and the family's functioning. It may also interfere with the process of grieving the loss of a "normal child," a necessary step toward facilitating an effective relationship with a child with a DD.

Several other stressors occur once DD has been diagnosed. People with DD and their families must begin to cope with the many differences between themselves and other families. The mantle of disability carries stigmatizing factors such as appearance, behavior, exclusion from typical daily routines and disruption of relationships by the special circumstances in which persons with DD and their families find themselves. Despite our commitment to a philosophy of viewing people with disabilities as people first, and as otherwise able, it will be some time before all of society accepts these views and accommodates individuals in a truly inclusive manner.

Family Stressors

When a person with a DD is also diagnosed with a mental disorder, this further burdens the individual and those caring for him or her. It generally means that they do not fit easily into either designated system and often have difficulty receiving necessary services. The dual diagnosis compounds the stigma because our society is not fully acceptant or tolerant of individuals with mental disorders. It also increases the caregivers' burden, not only because the individual is often more difficult to manage, but also because the families are saddened that the individual has not one but two disabling disorders. It may take a great deal of education and support for them to accept the mental disorder diagnosis.

Persons with DD and their families must also learn to cope with accessing and maintaining contact with the system or systems of services and supports that they need to promote habilitation. For many families, this is a daunting prospect fraught with fears: "Will my child receive the educational program that he or she needs before it is too late?" or "My child requires services not offered by his or her school…I know my rights, but how do I work with the system to assure that those services will be accessed?" or "I can't manage all of the appointments for services and supports needed by my child and still keep my job…who will help me?" There are no easy answers. The DD service system in most states and locales offers a wide range of services and supports, but many children require special, atypical options.

Transitions

The lives of persons with DD and their families are punctuated with difficult life transitions that begin in early childhood and extend throughout the lifespan. There are temporally and developmentally sequenced transition points such as home-to-school, school-to-work and work-to-retirement. These can have a significant impact on emotional and psychological development and the well being of the individual with DD. Those with ID also must cope with siblings surpassing them; isolation from peers, as the neighborhood children grow beyond them intellectually, and stigmatization by such things as riding on atypical transportation that usually announces the disability in the agency's name. This can lead to the development of disorders such as depression, dependent personality and anxiety. Non-sequenced transitions also occur, including health-to-illness, loss of a relative and residential re-location. All of these events may cause stress and precipitate disruptions in daily rhythms. Anticipation and appropriate interventions to prepare individuals and their families for such transitions are often very helpful.

OVERVIEW OF INTELLECTUAL DISABILITIES AND MENTAL DISORDERS
Historical Perspective

The history of individuals with ID reaches back to biblical times (Scheerenberger, 1982). Social isolation was a hallmark of society's response to persons with ID for nearly all of recorded history. During the Middle Ages, most persons with ID did not survive into adulthood and governments relied upon religious organizations to provide whatever care could not be supplied by families. In medieval times, many children with ID who survived infancy were placed in orphanages or simply sent out onto the street. The concept that care should be provided did not emerge until after the Period of Enlightenment (Scheerenberger, 1982). For all but a very few, someone other than the family assumed care-giving responsibility, usually in an institutional setting.

In the 1800 and 1900s, institutional care grew to be the primary residential alternative for people with ID. Initially operated by religious organizations, institutions grew in size and specificity and were gradually taken over by governmental units. By the early 1900s, over 200,000 Americans lived in such facilities (Scheerenberger, 1982). Initially, standards of care were high, and residents remained healthy, increasing survivorship into adulthood. However, as more and more families sought institutional care, costs rose and standard of care declined to the point where inhumane conditions widely existed (see Blatt and Kaplan's *Christmas in Purgatory, 1966,* for a stunning pictorial review of this slice of United States history). Only a very small number of persons with ID remained in community settings during this period. Among other things, neglect and lack of social structure in institutions gave rise to all the negative aspects of group dynamics, including the establishment of a hierarchical pecking order, competition for attention and behaviors such as aggression, non-compliance, and property destruction—not normally associated with a diagnosis of ID. Institutional responses to these behavior disturbances consisted largely of pharmacological treatment, physical restraint and further isolation.

During the 1960s, legal challenges to human rights compromises in institutions led to a historical reformation of care principles and strategies. Models developed and tested in Scandinavia that emphasized "normalization" of the life courses of individuals with disabilities (Wolfensberger, 1972) were widely disseminated in the United States. Legislative reform of public laws governing the financing of services to persons with disabilities mandated a shift from institutional to community-based and family-centered care. By the 1990s, most U.S. states had either fully closed or substantially reduced the census of their institutions (Braddock, Hemp, Parrish, & Westrich, 1998). Community alternatives to institutional care proliferated and inclusive services and supports were mandated by numerous U.S. federal laws, including the Developmental Disabilities Bill of Rights and Assistance Act, the Social Security Act, the Rehabilitation Act, the Individuals with Disabilities Education Act (IDEA) and the Americans with Disabilities Act (ADA).

These public policy and legislative efforts have resulted in elaboration of a full spectrum of publicly financed, highly individualized, educational, habilitative and family support services as well as small group and individual living arrangements. Infant mortality and health care have improved to the point where survival into older adulthood among persons with ID is very similar to survivorship among the non-disabled population. Institutional care is now not an option for most persons with ID in the United States (Braddock et al., 1998).

Wide ranges of mental disorders occur at least as often in persons with ID as in non-disabled persons (Davidson, Janicki, & Prasher, 2003; Thorpe, Davidson, & Janicki, 2000). However, this was not recognized until recently. Throughout most of recorded history, there was no differentiation between individuals with ID and concomitant mental disorders. Ideas as to the causes of these disorders ("afflictions") paralleled societal beliefs and over the ages individuals with ID were characterized as being possessed, divine, sinful, diseased, or immoral depending upon what was in vogue. Treatment also closely followed societal values—cycling between humanistic care and exclusion from society. With the latter, very abusive treatment often occurred, followed by responses to reform and protect. At times people with ID were tortured, raped, hunted as witches, used as slave labor or physically abused; at other times they were thought to have divine powers and even worshipped.

At the end of the 18th century the ideals of Romanticism, which expressed a love of nature and all things natural, and the intellectual climate of the Enlightenment influenced care of those with ID, as a wave of humanitarianism began to rise throughout Europe. In 1792 when Phillipe Pinel became director of the Bicêtre, the large mental institution in Paris, he "cast off the chains of the insane" (Mora, 1980). He believed these individuals were diseased, not sinful or immoral. He stressed the use of moral treatment: kindness rather than punishment. At the beginning of the 19th century, Pinel and the French physician Jean-Marc Gaspard Itard became catalysts for scientific study and professional concern with "idiocy" (Rosen, Clark, & Kivitz, 1976). When a teenage boy was found living in the woods and brought to Itard, who was working with deaf and blind individuals, he attempted to use both habilitative and therapeutic techniques to socialize and educate this "Wild Boy of Aveyron" (Harrison, 1980). Though he was unsuccessful, he passed on his ideas to a young psychiatrist, also working in Paris, named Edouard Seguin. In 1838, a school for "idiots," the term used at that time to describe those with ID, opened in Paris at the Salpetriere, and Seguin became its director. He also published the first work on the effectiveness of systematic training with individuals with ID, "*Traitement Moral, Hygiene et Education des Idiots [Moral Treatment, Hygiene and Education of Idiots]*" (Tredgold, 1937). Facilities now begun to develop throughout Europe: in Germany by Saegert and Kern, in Switzerland by Guggenbuhl and in England by Andrew Reed. People like these influenced Benjamin Rush and Dorothea Dix as they worked in America for development of more humanistic care (Feigelson, 1980). In 1833, the Worchester State Hospital in Massachusetts opened as the prototype of the modern American state mental hospital. Soon other, mental hospitals and schools for the "idiotic and feebleminded" opened throughout the Northeast and the Midwest (Rosen et al., 1976) and were influenced by Seguin's work (Rosen et al., 1976).

Distinctions between mental disorders and ID began to emerge in the last half of the 19th century. Some suggested that idiocy resulted from a lack of education or was due to

---

BOX 1.1
Terms Used in the 19th and Early 20th Centuries (From Penrose, 1934 & Tredgold, 1937)

Idiots — Persons in whose case there exists mental defectiveness of such a degree that they are unable to guard themselves against common physical dangers.

Imbeciles — Mental defectiveness which, though not amounting to idiocy, is yet so pronounced that they are incapable of managing themselves or their affairs or, in the case of children, of being taught to do so.

Feeble-Minded — Mental defectiveness which, though not amounting to imbecility, is yet so pronounced that they require care, supervision, and control for their own protection or for the protection of others, or, in the case of children, that they appear to be permanently incapable by reason of such defectiveness of receiving proper benefit from the instruction in ordinary schools.

Lunatic — Person who hath had understanding, but by disease, grief or other accident, hath lost the use of his reason.

Epileptics — A type of Amentia; arrest of neuronic development as an incidental phase in a degenerative process (which may be due to germ abnormality).

Morons — The "feeble-minded grade" in America (from the Greek word meaning "a fool - a person mainly lacking in judgment and good sense").

Mental Defective — Mental defectiveness coupled with strongly vicious or criminal propensities, and who require care, supervision and control for the protection of others [*And in Act quoted*] means a condition of arrested or incomplete development of mind existing before the age of eighteen years, whether arising from inherent causes or induced by disease or injury.

mental disorders. There were a number of somewhat crude methods of classifying mental disorders, including ID considered as dementia.

While debate about the causes, manifestations and classification of mental disorders, including epilepsy, continued, attempts were also being made to characterize the disorders. A number of terms were used in an attempt to delineate the differences (as shown in Box 1.1). Though these seem demeaning at present, they serve to show the evolution in thinking about the disorders.

In the late 1800s laws began to define the needs and prescribe certain treatments and methods of care for persons with ID and mental disorders within society (Scheerenberger, 1982). They led to the differentiation of care for individuals with "lunacy" (mental disorder) and those with mental deficiency (the term then used for ID). Separate institutional systems were established for the care of each group as well as their separation from society. During this time, however, many psychiatrists remained as directors of the institutions and continued to work with people with ID. When the American Association on Mental Deficiency was founded in 1876, all of its charter members were psychiatrists. They believed that psychotherapeutic principles and dynamically oriented education would be effective in "improving idiots and imbeciles."

This was to change at the end of the century when the Parisian School of Psychiatry and Neurology espoused the thesis of cerebral pathology. This led to various "defect theories," suggesting a limitation as to how much one could change these individuals, which further segregated the two groups. Additionally in the early 20th century the psychologist Alfred Binet and his student Theodore Simon developed a test that made the psychiatric assessment seemingly unnecessary for individuals with ID (Penrose, 1934). Their mental disability could be readily identified in terms of an Intelligence Quotient (IQ) and clearly indicate the future course of care.

The Binet IQ Test also led to the discovery of a large number of individuals who had mild ID and manifested socially unacceptable behaviors (Penrose, 1934), thus identifying a group threatening to the rest of society. The movement to protect the impaired and vulnerable individuals with ID and mental disorders soon became a movement *to remove them to protect society* as supported by Social Darwinism (survival of the fittest) in the early 20th century (Rosen et al., 1976) and the rise of Eugenics, the social policy that ensured the passing on of only the "best" genes. This development even further emphasized the need for "segregation of moral imbeciles" and thus the growth of larger institutions. At the same time psychiatry, in general, and American psychiatry, in particular, was immersed in the new concepts of psychoanalysis, a therapeutic intervention approach that excluded individuals with ID due to the beliefs that:

- Their inability to use abstract reasoning diminished their ability to examine their own behaviors, consider past causes and project into the future to imagine changes;

- They were unable to recognize that they had any responsibility for their behaviors or find reason to change them;

- They were unable to accurately recall past events, perform the mental functions of examining one's own behaviors and attempt to change them, or consider defense mechanisms.

There were also numerous beliefs as to why individuals with ID could not have mental disorders. It was thought that:
- They did not develop cognitively enough to regress, as was thought to be necessary for the diagnosis of Schizophrenia;
- They could not develop depression or low self esteem because their low intelligence kept them from experiencing their deficiencies (Szymanski, 1994);
- They could not experience attachments and therefore could not experience affect such as depression;
- Their ID protected them, and
- They could not inherit both a mental disorder and ID.

Contrary to these ideas, some people in the early 20th century believed that individuals with ID might actually be more susceptible to mental disorders, more vulnerable to stress and have fewer coping skills. Later studies have borne this out showing a prevalence rate of mental disorders in ID of anywhere from 20 to 40 % (Jacobson, in press).

Diagnostic overshadowing, the incorrect assumption that symptoms of frank mental disorders are within the range of behaviors normally associated with ID, resulted from the historical confusion of mental disorders in ID (Reiss, Levitan, & Szyszko, 1982). This further prevented practitioners from recognizing mental disorders in individuals with ID.

As the institutions for those with ID grew, the roles of the clinicians became stratified. Psychiatrists were no longer involved in most centers except occasionally as consultants. Psychologists began to fill the void left by the psychiatrists and, as there were no other adequate treatments, perfected their expertise in behavioral management. Social workers were social case managers, a role specifically defined as the interface between the doctor and the family. Their job was to gather pertinent history, schedule meetings, inform families about the care of their loved ones, and make arrangements for necessary services. Nurses carried out the traditional, institutional roles of ministering to the sick and ensuring that the residents received proper health care. As psychotropic medications became available, they were prescribed for the individuals with severe behavior disturbances to prevent serious injury to themselves and the staff. But because the belief held that individuals with ID could not have mental disorders, psychiatrists generally did not issue diagnoses of major mental disorders or specify treatment.

Additionally, another result of the institutional separation by IQ was the initiative across the U.S. to separate the state agencies as well as the funding for the two groups of clients. This precipitated definition of the concepts "primary disability," that is, the diagnosis, either ID or mental disorder, most likely responsible for the clinical status of the individual and that which determines the system of care, and "complete separation of care," that is, in mental health agencies or agencies for those with ID. As a result one system or the other excluded individuals based upon the criteria for admission. Skills and approaches varied greatly and staff generally was trained in only one theoretical approach. These factors created a wide divergence in the development of care for those individuals in the mental health system, particularly those in ID.

SERVICE ISSUES

Spectrum of Services

In general, states, territories and the federal government share responsibility for financing the ID service system in the U.S. Appropriations flowing from large federal programs such as Medicaid (Title XIX of the Social Security Act), the Rehabilitation Act and the Individuals with Disabilities Education Act (IDEA) are often matched by state governments to fund residential, day and special education services as well as to support a wide variety of other service options including respite, in-home programming, family support services, specialty clinic services, transportation and vocational rehabilitation. Both state and private voluntary agencies at the local level provide such services. Over the past 30 years, the spectra of options for major direct services (residential, day programs and special education) have expanded and increased in flexibility to the point where a high degree of individualization can be achieved. Most states have opted to participate in the Medicaid 1196 Waiver Program that allows providers to deliver only those services that a client and his or her family actually needs. The flexibility afforded by this program has proven valuable in addressing the needs of persons with clinical profiles such as those with mental disorders and ID.

Client Rights

A very important feature of the ID service system is its capacity to protect individual rights and to provide independent, individual, legal and systems advocacy when those rights are threatened or compromised. The Protection and Advocacy System, a national network of advocates funded by the Developmental Disabilities Bill of Rights and Assistance Act, carry out these functions within states. Each state implements this program differently, but the particular organization within each state designated to provide these services is always independent from all other state, local or private voluntary service agencies.

The Role of the Primary Health Care Provider

A primary health care provider should follow every person with ID. While medical concerns comprise only a small part of the clinical and habilitative service needs of people with ID, the medical provider is in a unique position to assist families in identifying service needs and facilitating access to them. Most importantly, the primary care provider can act as an advocate for the client and his or her family and assist caregivers in coordinating multiple services and supports. Specialists such as consulting psychiatrists and psychologists who serve consumers and their families may also function in these roles but must keep the primary care provider informed about their activities and seek his or her advice about changes in the service plan.

Service Coordination/Case Management

Almost every person with ID will require individualized services and supports tailored to his or her needs and preferences. Consumers and their families are always mandatory participants in the planning for those services and supports. Nearly always the plan will require coordination, since individual services in the plan may be derived from more than one provider. Service coordination is an important component of the service system in the U.S. Free of charge, it provides each client with a person with expertise in services coordination. The service coordinator/case manager may serve as the client's advocate and assist them in accessing or changing services, arranging for transportation, completing required forms for benefits and acting as a liaison between the client and his or her family and their community providers.

Special issues

Persons with mental disorders and ID may have to access services and support from two different systems: one that offers ID services and the other that offers mental health services. Coordinating these different services may be difficult. In the case of children, this may fall to the parent, the child's best advocate, who may lack sufficient knowledge and energy to navigate the boundaries between systems. Persons with mental disorders and ID and their families often require a complex and diverse mix of services and supports. Accessing and maintaining these services may require extraordinary vigilance and persistence. The most difficult challenge tends to be retaining clinically appropriate services from the mental health system. There is a shortage of psychiatrists and other mental health professionals with expertise in diagnosing and treating mental disorders in clients with ID. Documenting eligibility for mental health services may vary in difficulty from locale to locale, complicating timely access to the ideal array of specialized services to prevent loss of primary placement and basic habilitative services.

In general, the ID service system in the U.S. has vastly improved over the past half-century since institutional care has been replaced with community inclusion. However, the system still does not respond well universally to individuals with complex needs and calls for much more attention to these aspects of service.

SUMMARY

Over recent years, though we have witnessed the emergence of advances in the understanding of the etiology, diagnosis, treatment and models of service for people having both conditions of ID and mental disorder, individuals with ID and mental disorders still have difficulty getting the care that they need. Public policy has generally mirrored social policy. Both have had enormous impact upon the labeling and care of individuals with ID and mental disorders. Each greatly influences the funding for and accessibility to programs and care for persons who are differently able. Numerous forces over the past century separated the care of individuals with ID from those with mental disorders, leading to a complete separation in thinking about the disorders. This situation has resulted in a lack of understanding at all levels about the occurrence and presentation of mental disorders in individuals with ID. The movement to keep individuals with ID in their communities, to enhance their innate abilities and to recognize their rights as individuals has helped to change this. However, history reveals that this can deteriorate quickly. Individuals with mental disorders or ID can easily become marginalized and lose support for necessary care and services. This can be compounded for those with both disorders. It will be an ongoing challenge for clients and providers to continue to advocate for well-informed, cost effective, quality services that combine expertise in mental disorders and ID.

REFERENCES

AAMR (2002). *Mental retardation: Definition, classification, and systems of support* (10th ed.). Washington, DC: American Association on Mental Retardation.

American Psychiatric Association (2000). *Diagnostic and statistical manual of mental disorders* (Rev. 4th ed.). Washington, DC: American Psychiatric Association.

Batshaw, M. (2002). *Chromosomes and heredity: A toss of the dice*. In M. Batshaw (Ed.), *Children with Disabilities* (5th ed., pp. 3-26). Baltimore: Brookes Publishing Co.

Batshaw, M., & Shapiro, B. (2002). Intellectual disabilities. In M. Batshaw (Ed.), *Children with Disabilities* (5th ed., pp. 287-306). Baltimore: Brookes Publishing Co.

Black, S.A. (1999). Cerebral Palsy. In M. Levine, W. Carey, & A. Crocker (Eds.), *Developmental-behavioral pediatrics* (3th ed., pp. 579-588). Philadelphia: W. B. Saunders.

Blatt, B., & Kaplan, F. (1966). *Christmas in purgatory*. Boston: Allyn, & Bacon.

Braddock, D., Hemp, R., Parish, S., & Westrich, J. (1998). *The state of the states in developmental disabilities* (5th ed.). Washington, DC: American Association on Intellectual Disabilities.

Crocker, A. C. (1987). The spectrum of medical care for developmental disabilities. In I. L. Rubin & A .C. Crocker (Eds.). *Developmental disabilities: Delivery of medical care for children and adults* (pp. 10-22). Philadelphia: Lea & Febiger.

Davidson, P. W., Janicki, M. P., & Prasher, V. P. (2003) Introduction: Aging, intellectual disability, and emotional and behavioral health. In P. W. Davidson, V. P. Prasher, & M. P. Janicki (Eds.), *Mental health, intellectual disabilities and the aging process* (pp. 1-6). Oxford, England: Blackwell Science.

Feigelson, E. B. (1980). Hospitalization and milieu therapy. In H. I. Kaplan, A. M. Freedman, & B. J. Sadock (Eds.), *Comprehensive textbook of psychiatry* Vol. 3. Baltimore: Williams & Wilkins Co.

Harrison, S. I. (1980). Child Psychiatry: Psychiatric Treatment. In H. I. Kaplan, A. M. Freedman, & B. J. Sadock (Eds.), *Comprehensive textbook of psychiatry* Vol. 3. Baltimore: Williams & Wilkins Co.

Jacobson, J. & Mulick, J. (1995) (Eds.), *Manual of diagnostic and professional practice in mental retardation*. Washington, DC: American Psychological Association.

Levy, S. (1996). The developmental disabilities. In L. Kurtz, P. Dowrick, S. Levy, & M. Batshaw (Eds.), *Handbook of developmental disabilities: Resources for interdicisplinary care* (pp. 3-11). Gaithersburg, MD: Aspen Publishers.

Mora, G. (1980) Historical and Theoretical Trends in Psychiatry. In H. I. Kaplan, A. M. Freedman, & B. J. Sadock (Eds.), *Comprehensive textbook of psychiatry* Vol. 3. Baltimore: Williams & Wilkins Co.

Penrose, L. S., (1934). *Mental defect*. New York: Farrar & Rinehart.

Reiss, S., Levitan, G. W., Szyszko, J. (1982) Emotional disturbance and mental retardation: Diagnostic overshadowing, *American Journal of Mental Deficiency, 86,* 567-574.

Rosen, M., Clark, G. R., & Kivitz, M. S. (1976) *The history of intellectual disabilities* Vol. 1: Collected papers. Baltimore: University Park Press.

Scheerenberger, R. (1982). *A history of intellectual disabilities*. Baltimore: Brookes Publishing Co.

Scheerenberger, R. (1987). *A history of intellectual disabilities: A quarter century of promise.* Baltimore: Brookes Publishing Co.

Szymanski, L. S. (1994). Intellectual disabilities and mental health: Concepts, aetiology and incidence. In N. Bouras, *Mental health in intellectual disabilities: Recent advances and practices.* Cambridge University Press.

Thorpe, L., Davidson, P., & Janicki, M. P. (2000). *Healthy aging - adults with intellectual disabilities: Biobehavioral issues.* Geneva, Switzerland: World Health Organization.

Tredgold, A. F. (1937). *Mental deficiency* (6th ed.). Baltimore: William Wood and Company.

WHO (1992). *The international classification of diseases and related health problems* (10th ed.). Geneva, Switzerland: World Health Organization.

Wolfensberger, W. (1972). *The principle of normalization in human services.* Toronto, Canada: National Institute on Intellectual Disabilities.

Assessment of Mental Disorders in Individuals with Intellectual Disability

John C. Pomeroy

INTRODUCTION

The diagnosis of mental disorders in persons with ID can be both complex and controversial. There is potential for a narrow biomedical approach to assessment that can lead to rapid use (or overuse) of pharmacotherapy without considering the multiple factors that may impact on the individual. Alternatively, the failure to accurately diagnose a treatable mental disorder can lead to prolonged suffering, distress and exposure to ineffective therapies. Good practice dictates that the assessment of individuals suspected of having both a mental disorder and ID requires careful analysis of all aspects of the individual and his or her environment. The foundation for such assessment is best exemplified by the concept of the biopsychosocial model that was first proposed by Engel (1977). Many workers in this field have used similar approaches adapted to their own models of assessment and treatment (e.g., Gardner & Sovner, 1994; Gardner & Whalen, 1996; Nezu, Nezu, & Gill-Weiss, 1992). This chapter will detail the importance of using the biopsychosocial model in assessment of mental disorders in people with ID.

Sovner and Hurley (1999) emphasize that a number of myths (shown in Table 2.1) related to this clinical area not only still exist but also are often ingrained in institutional policies.

ASSESSMENT APPROACHES AND GOALS

The assessment of mental disorder in the presence of ID is often completed in a number of stages. It usually begins with interviews with referrers and caregivers about presenting concerns. Subsequently, and in a sequence that may be determined by the acuity of need, there should be a gathering of history and past observations from multiple sources, including the review of all relevant available records as well as the direct observation, interview and assessment of the referred individual and their environment. Numerous other evaluations may be indicated, for example, medical assessment and behavioral analysis,

before reaching conclusions about diagnosis and treatment. The ultimate success of any evaluation will require:
- Integration of all of the material acquired from these many sources of information;
- A formulation that incorporates the multiple aspects of the assessment into a coherent summary of the probable cause or causes of the presenting problem, and
- The incorporation of this formulation into a more concise multi-axial diagnostic structure within which all aspects of the individual, and their environment, are addressed.

This process of systematic evaluation and conceptualization of the varied aspects of the individual should provide the framework for treatment decisions and ensure that each aspect of the biological, psychological and social factors are addressed either simultaneously or in sequence with the most acute issues being addressed first.

There are many formats that have been developed to ensure a comprehensive diagnostic process. In assessing mental disorders in the U.S., a five-axial, biopsychosocial approach developed and published by the American Psychiatric Association, the Diagnostic and Statistical Manual of Mental Disorders, Fourth Edition (DSM-IV-TR, APA 2000) is used by psychiatrists and most other mental health providers. On Axis I, the major mental disorders (e.g., Major Depressive Disorder, Generalized Anxiety Disorder) are recorded. More than one disorder may be present and multiple diagnoses may be recorded. Axis II records the level of ID (Mild to Profound Mental Retardation continues to be the terminology used in the DSM manual) and any diagnoses of Personality Disorder (e.g., Schizoid Personality Disorder, Borderline Personality Disorder). Axis III records major medical disorders (e.g., Diabetes, Hyperthyroidism). Axis IV documents significant social, occupational and

TABLE 2.1
Myths Regarding Behavior Disturbances and Mental Disorders*

Myth 1. Behavior always has functional significance and is under the control of the affected individual.
Myth 2. If a behavior has functional significance, it is unlikely to be related to a mental disorder.
Myth 3. A person with severe or profound disabilities is too impaired to develop classic mental disorders.
Myth 4. Bizarre behaviors, such as talking to oneself out loud, fantasy play or talking to an imaginary friend, always represent manifestations of psychosis.
Myth 5. Drug therapy is a restrictive form of behavior control. All regimens must, therefore, include a behavior plan and a timetable for discontinuing treatment.

* From Sovner & Hurley, 1999

environmental issues. The last, Axis V, is used to record the present level of functioning (psychological, social, and occupational) with an emphasis on the degree to which the symptoms of the mental disorder affect the individual's daily performance. A standardized scale, the Global Assessment of Functioning (GAF) Scale, which codes function from 0 to 100 and provides clinical descriptors of typical characteristics at each functional level, is commonly used for this axis. The use of this axis creates particular complications for assessment of individuals with ID, as it is unclear to what degree any functional difficulty that is primarily due to the ID should be incorporated into the rating. For example, significant occupational problems may always be present in many individuals with ID but the additional mental disorder may exacerbate problems in vocational or occupational settings and the GAF coding system does not factor in baseline functioning when providing a global assessment rating. Although not always ideal for some of the complex problems that are assessed in the area of mental disorders and ID, this approach, if used properly, provides a relatively comprehensive description of the clinical and diagnostic issues.

Other interesting models derived from the field of ID take a problem definition/problem-solving approach. Thus, from initial definition of the referral behavior (e.g., aggression, self-injury) the assessment information is evaluated and in varied structural approaches inserted into a visual problem-solving chart. This approach incorporates a diagnostic component but accentuates the multiple interplay of factors (e.g., client, care-giving system, and the environment, (Nezu et al., 1992). In addition, the complexity of the instigating and maintaining factors for the problem behaviors is considered from a biopsychosocial perspective (Gardner et al., 1994; Gardner et al., 1996). The visual charts that document the problems and necessary further assessment or intervention can ensure that each potential cause or exacerbating factor is addressed in a sequence that takes into account the priority of need. Such an approach is not so clearly addressed in the descriptive DSM-IV-TR model, as there is no defined hierarchy of the relative importance of each axis with regard to etiology and treatment priorities. This could lead to overemphasis on Axis I, the major mental disorder, as the focus of treatment intervention.

Most importantly, whatever specific conceptual structure is used, the assessment must ultimately document all aspects of the individual's social, biological, emotional, behavioral and psychological functioning along with the evidence for specific mental disorders as well as the other environmental and life circumstances that may be impacting the manifestation of the mental disorder.

THE ASSESSMENT MODEL OF MENTAL DISORDERS WITH INTELLECTUAL DISABILITIES

Traditionally the process of making the psychiatric diagnosis of a mental disorder has tended to accentuate categorical approaches based on cross-sectional evaluation of individuals at the specific time of presentation. This can lead to a narrow concept that merely defines the presence or absence of a specific condition or disorder, without taking into account the many variables that impact individuals and that may lead to the emergence of emotional and/or behavioral problems. Behavior can be a consequence of many factors. Given the difficulties in communication and cognition of individuals with ID, there is often a limited behavioral repertoire available to express many different types of distress. The assessment should consider the multiple influences and sources of stress on the manifestation of problem behaviors. These may relate to cognitive functioning, psychological issues, social and emotional influences, environmental factors and biomedical disorders. None of these aspects of the evaluation are mutually exclusive, as, for example, symptomatology

---

BOX 2.1

Biomedical Factors Influencing the Symptomatology of Mental Disorders

The medical factors that impact on the individual with mental disorders and ID could be considered from a number of perspectives:

Etiological (e.g., genetic, chromosomal, traumatic, infectious)
- ID research identifies more than 350 different causes, which can be subdivided into pre-, peri-, and post-natal, and include genetic chromosomal, infectious, biological-environmental and traumatic etiologies.
- Independent factors (i.e., they do not impact on the presentation of psychiatric symptomatology).
- Directly support a presentation of psychiatric symptomatology (e.g., behavioral phenotypes).

Associated Medical Condition
- Medical condition commonly associated with a particular syndrome that might impact on clinical presentation (e.g., sensory disorder in congenital rubella).
- General medical condition, which causes pain or discomfort, that may cause presentation of emotional/behavioral problems.
- Commonly associated medical/neurological disorders (e.g., seizures) that could influence the symptoms of a mental disorder.
- Medical disorder that may present as a mental disorder (e.g., thyroid disease, systemic lupus erythematosus).
- Symptoms of a mental disorder induced by medical treatments, particularly medication side effects.

Specific Medical Issues
- Certain syndromes can have broad physical effects impacting on anatomical characteristics or physiologic functioning (e.g., risk of thyroid disorder and/or heart disease in Down syndrome). Not only can these medical conditions provide physical morbidity, they can have an impact on emotional and behavioral health.

Medical Disorders that Mimic Mental Disorders
- Some medical disorders present with symptoms that are similar to mental disorders. Examples include: Hyperthyroidism with behaviors that can look like anxiety or mania, and Hypothyroidism that can slow down an individual and causes a clinical picture that may be indistinguishable from major depression.

Medications Can Cause Symptoms of Mental Disorders
- Examples are antidepressants that can speed up an individual and look like mania or cause a feeling of anxiety, and propranolol, which can cause the symptoms of depression.

may be a consequence of a specific mental disorder but the presenting characteristics may be highly influenced (exacerbated or ameliorated) by other factors that are revealed by the broader assessment. Therefore, the crucial aspects of assessment are related not only to accurate evaluation of individual factors but also to all of these factors.

Biomedical Factors

Behavioral and emotional problems observed in individuals with ID could be a consequence of biomedical factors through numerous mechanisms, as briefly outlined in Box 2.1. Undiagnosed medical conditions can contribute to or present as mental disorders and behavior disorders. In one study (Ryan & Sunada, 1997) it was found that up to 75% of individuals with ID being assessed for mental disorders had previously misdiagnosed or under-treated medical conditions. Nearly half of these individuals were receiving medications that could produce symptoms like those of mental disorders.

The medical assessment is a crucial aspect of the evaluation of individuals with mental disorders and ID. The clinician should differentiate between that part of the assessment that focuses on the biomedical etiology of the ID (e.g., investigation for an underlying genetic

TABLE 2.2
Factors Influencing Emotional or Behavioral Disturbances: Utilizing a Biopsychosocial Model

Biomedical	Psychosocial/Environmental
• Medical disorders causing pain or discomfort (e.g., middle ear infection, dental pain) • Medical disorders presenting with symptoms of mental disorders (e.g., Thyroid disorder, Wilson's Disease) • Sensory impairments • Negative side effects of medication (e.g., akathisia due to neuroleptics) • Allergies • Seizure disorder • Constipation • Sleep disturbance • Nutritional deficiencies • Use of caffeine or nicotine	• Noxious stimuli in the home or work place • Abuse • Problems with peers • Environmental changes • Family dysfunction • Inappropriate expectations from staff/caregivers • Controlling/inflexible environment
Life Events *Childhood* • Effects of initial diagnosis • Starting school • Sibling issues – new baby, comparing skills, etc. • Puberty/adolescence • Sexuality/dating • Leaving school/"Aging Out"	**Life Events** *Adulthood* • Changes in residence and staff • Relating to new caregivers and peers • Reducing or not meeting expectations • Intimate relationships • Losses – parents, relatives • Aging • Physical changes and medical issues

syndrome), and the assessment of other medical conditions that may be active and impacting the individual's behavior. Extensive investigation for neurobiological causation using tools such as, MRIs or EEGs, is usually of limited value unless clinical characteristics (e.g., physical anomalies, skin lesions and seizures) are suggestive of a specific biologic cause. Careful review of bodily systems by history and examination should guide the clinician to rational approaches to further investigation.

Psychosocial Factors

Often behavior disorders in people with ID are an immediate reaction to stressors in the environment. There should always be an attempt to identify environmental factors that can explain behaviors and should be modified as part of the client's treatment plan (See Table 2.2).

Psychological issues that impact on individuals with ID are numerous and could be viewed from a number of perspectives. One useful life-span model considers the impact of the cognitive limitations on management of stress with particular emphasis on the predictable life events that could create stress for a typical individual with ID (Levitas & Gilson, 2001). This model observes that many individuals with ID have difficulty in coping with situations that call for novel responses and increased independence. Even expected events can become stressful and rapidly advance from stressor to cause of a behavior disorder. With knowledge of the events that could precipitate a perceived crisis, (see Table 2.2) accurate interpretation of the likely etiology and nature of the emotional distress could lead to more appropriate intervention. In the early years of the life of the individual with ID, many of the potential developmental problems are related to challenges due to the ID or awareness of the limitations associated with ID on the life of the child or adolescent and the family. In adulthood, the presentation of problems are typically due to challenges in adaptive skills and independent functioning—demands that may be beyond the individual's level of comfort. In addition, there are some critical events that could occur at any time of life and would be traumatic events for anyone but could further undermine the self-confidence of the individual with ID. (See Chapter 1.)

In the evaluation stage it is important to remember that children and adults with ID are at significant risk of physical and sexual abuse (Ammerman, Hersen, VanHasselt, Lubetsky, & Sieck, 1994; Turk & Brown, 1994). The true prevalence of abuse remains unknown but maltreatment may initiate or exacerbate behavioral and emotional disturbance. The potential for abuse can also occur in the context of a mental disorder when caregivers engage in inappropriate physical interactions in response to the disruptive behavior of the individual. It is not clear that abuse leads to any specific patterns of mental disorders but some literature (e.g., Haaven, Little, & Petrie-Miller, 1990) would suggest that sexual abuse could increase the risk of an individual later engaging in sex offenses against others.

Special Issues in the Assessment of Mental Disorders in the Presence of ID

Certain features of the communication and behavior of individuals with ID may confuse the examiner in assessing for the presence of symptoms of mental disorders. Table 2.3 describes a number of common situations, which, if ignored, can lead to error in the assessment of mental disorders and behavior disorders in individuals with ID. Developmentally appropriate behavior in adults with ID may resemble symptoms of mental disorders in

Table 2.3
*Potential Causes of Error in Diagnosing Mental Disorders in the Presence of ID**

Intellectual Distortion: Misinterprests unusual speech or thought processes as psychotic or reflecting emotional disturbance when actually due to poor cognitive and communication skills.

Psychosocial Masking: Observer lacks awareness of the world of those with ID causing misunderstanding of true symptoms of a mental disorder (e.g., a grandiose idea of a manic individual may be to assert the ability to live alone or drive a car).

Cognitive Disintegration: Under stress individuals with ID may have extreme reactions that are interpreted as psychotic or due to severe disturbance but merely reflect acute, stress-related adjustment problems.

Baseline Exaggeration: Mental Disorders can sometimes present as an exacerbation of behavior that is also seen in the baseline state (e.g., the occasionally aggressive individual who becomes excessively aggressive during a depressive illness).

* **Summarized from Sovner & Hurley, 1989**

non-disabled persons of the same chronological age. Thus, accurate interpretation of such behaviors as self-talking, agitation under stress, disorganization and stereotypies is complicated by the fact that these may be normal behaviors for this individual, taking into account developmental and cognitive levels. Alternatively, these characteristics may be secondary to biological, neurological or environmental factors and unrelated to any frank psychopathology. However, in some cases these behaviors could actually be due to underlying disorders of thought, mood, anxiety or other mental disorders.

In comparison with typically developing individuals, those with ID who have true mental disorders may present with unusual or atypical symptoms. For example, an exacerbation of self-injury or stereotypies may be the presenting concern that is actually due to the emergence of a specific mental disorder such as depression or anxiety. Lack of communication skills often prevents clarification of feelings and thoughts that would usually be elicited by psychiatric interview. Observation of behavior may be the only clue to the presence of a mental disorder. Situational variation in presentation among individuals with mental disorders and ID is also common, and symptoms may not manifest themselves in the same way at home, at work or in the treatment setting. The clinician often must rely on staff or caregiver reports that may be imprecise or inaccurate. Despite these concerns, mental disorders commonly present in individuals with ID essentially as described in current diagnostic manuals (e.g., DSM-IV-TR, APA, 2000) or the International Classification of Psychiatric and Behavioral Disorders, 10th Edition, ICD-10 (WHO, 1992), particularly in persons with stronger intellectual and communication abilities.

The World Health Organization (1996) has produced an adaptation of the ICD-10 diagnostic manual for individuals with ID. However, an early trial of the manual invoked some criticisms regarding such aspects as the content of specific axes and the validity of some specific (often single symptom) diagnoses and their diagnostic criteria (Einfeld & Tonge, 1999). No adaptation of DSM-IV-TR has been developed. Interesting discussion of the practical utilization of Axes IV and V in the presence of ID has been initiated (Hurley, 2001), specifically addressing the need to differentiate between those functional difficulties that are related to the mental disorders and those due to ID.

Accurate and valid diagnosis of mental disorders in individuals with ID often requires assessment of emotional and behavioral patterns over time. Paying attention to more objective clinical signs such as sleep, appetite, weight and activity-level change is particularly important (See Box 2.2). Evidence of an onset of change and patterns of recurrence or cyclicity of problems can be a useful indicator of an underlying mental disorder. Individuals with mental disorders and ID may manifest sudden or significant changes in adaptive daily living skills or functional behavior at work or home. Such a change may have occurred at a time more remote than recognized by those providing the history. It is crucial that assessors obtain a detailed developmental and past history; symptoms that may be due to chronic mental disorders (e.g., schizophrenia) could have become considered the individual's usual way of being.

BOX 2.2
Behavioral Characteristics that Raise Suspicion of Mental Disorder
- Behavior disturbances that occur across all settings.
- Behavior disturbances that do not respond to well-designed consistent behavioral intervention and habilitative programming.
- Behavior disturbances that are associated with concurrent changes in sleep, appetite, sexual activity and/or daily functioning.
- Evidence of hyper-arousal with increased autonomic activity (e.g., tremors, fast pulse, sweating) accompanying the behaviors.

Any of these, in addition to other evidence, could assist in making an appropriate treatment decision.

Disorders such as mood disorders, severe anxiety, schizophrenia or other psychoses are nearly always associated with decline in daily living and work skills, and an increase in socially inappropriate behaviors at some point in the individual's life. However, many other factors could also cause such functional deterioration, and it is important to complete a functional behavioral analysis to evaluate environmental stimuli or individual characteristics that might have initiated or reinforced behavior disturbances. There are few "symptoms" that are specific to mental disorders. Some hints (See Box 2.2) regarding when to consider an independent mental disorder might be identified in the course of a behavioral analysis.

An important, relatively new, approach to studying the interaction between ID and the manifestation of behavior disturbances has focused on behavioral phenotypes. Certain well-defined syndromes due to known genetic or chromosomal abnormalities have been found to be associated with behavioral characteristics that are observed relatively consistently among groups of individuals with the same etiology. Down syndrome, Fragile-X, Prader-Willi, Cornelia de Lange and Lesch-Nyhan syndromes are typically associated with specific patterns of behaviors or symptoms that have been called behavioral phenotypes. For example, behaviors such as aggression, withdrawal or self-injury commonly accompany the Lesch-Nyhan and Cornelia de Lange syndromes. Depression and dementia may occur in older people with Down syndrome. It is hoped that this knowledge will lead to improved understanding of the neurobiological mechanisms that may underlie the relationship between genetically determined neurobiological variations and the manifestation of specific behavioral characteristics.

THE ASSESSMENT

A thorough evaluation will require a number of steps (See Box 2.3). The evaluation usually utilizes a team of professionals from different disciplines (e.g., psychology, psychiatry, neurology, social work), ideally coordinated and managed by one particular team leader, who may be from any of the involved disciplines, but should be able to understand and integrate the multiple sources of information. The team leader will coordinate the members of the team, ensuring that a timely and thorough evaluation is completed, and that necessary interventions are initiated based on the conclusions of the team.

BOX 2.3
Elements of a Comprehensive Evaluation/Assessment

For individuals with ID a thorough approach to assessment for mental disorders should include:
- **Initial Consultation:** Clearly define referral problems and specific difficulties, obtain past history (including birth and developmental history, initial examples of behavior and treatment history) and gather family psychiatric history.
- **Evaluation of strengths and deficits:** Secure psychological testing, adaptive behavior profile and assessment of environmental factors.
- **Comprehensive medical assessment:** Secure medical and developmental history, physical examination, appropriate laboratory tests, as well as consultation with specialists such as neurologists, speech pathologists, audiologists and occupational therapists, as indicated.
- **Observational Analysis:** Complete mental status, clinical interview and functional analysis of behavior
- **Synthesis:** Synthesize information to develop a diagnostic formulation and initial treatment plan.

Initial Consultation

Individuals with mental disorders and ID may be unable to provide an accurate history of their developmental, clinical and treatment history. It is crucial that information is obtained from multiple sources (e.g., family, caregivers, teachers, trainers and administrators) and organized in a structured format that includes presenting symptoms, developmental history, review of physical systems, social history and present situation, previous medical and psychiatric treatment and caregiver attitudes and understanding. This should provide a thorough account of relevant past and present aspects of the referred individual's functioning. The availability of extensive past records can be crucial in developing a picture of both the individual's characteristic traits and the course and character of the apparent disorder. This is particularly true for adults who have been in care outside of their family of origin for long periods of time. It is important to have a clear structure to the history gathering process and to follow a consistent format with the aim of developing a life-history model that characterizes the individual. It should not be assumed that informants will know to tell the assessor the important and relevant information required; so specific questioning regarding symptoms and associated physiologic or behavioral changes is necessary.

Assessment Tools

As diagnosis of mental disorders has become more standardized and based on valid, reliable and measurable criteria, many approaches have been taken to develop diagnostic tools that can provide greater reliability, where assessors improve objectivity and better structure the assessment process.

These tools (See Tables 2.4a & b) include:
- Diagnostic interviews (with varying degrees of structure and clinical focus) that can be done with the identified individual and/or other informants;
- Psychometric scales and checklists (also completed by the identified client or observers) that can focus on a specific diagnosis, numerous aspects of behavior or general screening characteristics of mental disorders, and
- Standardized observational measures, particularly for situations where the identified client is unable to be assessed by formal interview.

Although many of the tools have been developed to aid diagnosis, their application is often more helpful in providing a methodology for objectively measuring change over time and/or response to treatment. While these tools should not be used as a sole source of information regarding clinical diagnoses, they can often ensure that all aspects of clinical inquiry are adequately addressed.

Since 1980, numerous scales and assessment tools, such as those listed in Tables 2.4a and 2.4b, have been developed for assessing mental disorders and behavior disorders in the presence of ID. Less commonly, standardized general-use diagnostic interviews or self-report rating scales have been usefully applied to those with mental disorders and ID, mostly in individuals with mild ID (e.g., Zung Depression Rating Scale - Burt, Loveland, & Lewis, 1992: SADS-L Diagnostic Interview - Meadows et al., 1991).

When using these tools, the clinician needs to be aware of the most appropriate application (i.e., a diagnostic instrument or behavioral rating scale) and the strengths and weaknesses of the measure. For example, the commonly used Aberrant Behavior Checklist (ABC) (Aman & Singh, 1986) completed by an observer, provides a comprehensive range of potential behavioral disturbances that can be reduced to scores on five empirically derived factors. Many clinicians will use this measure as an initial guide, but it may prove to be a more useful measure of treatment response or change over time when completed on a regular basis during the intervention/treatment phase. Some scales are more appropriate for different levels of functioning (e.g., Diagnostic Assessment of the Severely Handicapped (DASH) Scale for adults with severe to profound ID (Matson, Gardner, Coe, & Sovner, 1991) or different age groups. Some are focused more on general behavior whereas others attempt to address the diagnostic constructs of mental disorders. Tables 2.4a and 2.4b provide a brief indication for each assessment measure listed.

TABLE 2.4a
Commonly Used Scales and Interview Formats: Mental Disorders and ID

Aberrant Behavior Checklist (ages six and up): 58-item informant rating scale with five sub-scales derived from factor analysis. (Aman & Singh, 1986, 1994)

AAMR Adaptive Behavior Scale – Second Edition: Maladaptive behavior ratings in 14 domains covering a large number of behaviors on three-point scale. (Nihira, Leland & Lambert, 1993)

DASH (Diagnostic Assessment of the Severely Handicapped) (Adults): 96-item informant rating scale tied to DSM-IV-TR diagnostic structure for use with adults with severe to profound ID. (Matson, Coe, Gardner & Sovner, 1991)

Developmental Behavior Checklist (ages four and up): Based on the Child and Behavior Checklist with forms for caregiver and teacher. Sub-scales derived by factor analysis. (Einfeld & Tonge, 1994)

Emotional Problems Scales (Adolescents and Adults): Informant rating and self-rating scales. Intended for individuals with borderline to mild ID. 12 sub-scales on informant scale and six sub-scales (including a lie scale) on self-report. (Strohmer & Prout, 1991)

PIIDA (Adults) 56 items on both informant rating and self-rating scales. Intended to be based on interview. Scales approximate eight major psychiatric diagnostic groups and are useful for screening. (Matson, 1997)

Reiss Screen for Maladaptive Behavior (ages 12 and up): 38-item scale completed by caregivers. Used for full range of ID. Good instrument to measure response to treatment. (Reiss, 1988)

Reiss Scale for Children's Psychiatric Disorders and ID (Children and Adolescents): Similar to Reiss Screen. Covers problematic childhood behaviors. (Reiss & Valenti-Hein, 1994)

Psychiatric Assessment Schedule for Adults with Developmental Disability (PAS-ADD): A diagnostic interview for psychiatrists to assess people with ID. (Moss et al., 1993)

The PAS-ADD Checklist: A screening instrument for use by care staff to detect mental health problems in adults with ID. (Moss et. el., 1998)

The MINI PAS-ADD: An assessment schedule for use by health professionals to detect mental health problems in adults with ID. (Moss, 2001)

Assessment of Cognitive, Communication and Adaptive Skills

These three areas of functioning may be impacted as a consequence of the ID as well as mental disorders. Functional limitations may in turn cause behavioral disturbances that may mimic symptoms of mental disorders. In establishing diagnoses, developmental causes for functional deficits must be distinguished from those caused by mental disorders.

TABLE 2.4b   *Commonly Used Scales & Interview Formats: Autism and Pervasive Developmental Disorder*
Autism Behavior Checklist: 57-item observer-screening checklist in five areas of functioning. Not a diagnostic instrument but good for measuring treatment effects. (Krug, Arick & Almond, 1980)
CARS Observational rating scale: May over-identify Autism in the presence of language impairment and moderate to severe ID. Reliable screening instrument (Schopler, Reichler & Renner, 1988)
ADI-R: Semi-structured investigator-based interview of caregivers. Linked to current diagnostic systems. Requires training and standardization; full and shortened versions. Presently the gold standard for diagnosis of Autism when combined with the ADOS-G. (Lord, Rutter & LeCouter, 1994)
ADOS-G: Standardized protocol for observation of social and communicative skills of children suspected of having Autism/PDD. Requires standardized training. (DiLavore, Lord, & Rutter, 1999)

A comprehensive evaluation should include, as deemed appropriate by the team:
- Assessment of communicative functions, including expressive and receptive languageskills and auditory processing deficits (Speech Pathology, Audiology);
- Neurocognitive assessment, including an estimate of general cognitive ability as well as tests of specific cognitive functions such as attention, memory, executive functions, and reaction time (Psychology), and
- Evaluation of social and adaptive behavior, including skills of daily living and social adaptation (Social Work, Psychology).

The goal of these evaluations is not only to identify relative limitations but also to highlight strengths that may become an important component of positive intervention.

Medical Assessment

The components of the medical examination of an individual with a mental disorder and ID are essentially the same and should be given to any individual presenting symptoms of a mental disorder, paying greater attention to the likelihood that the individual cannot give specific information regarding their symptomatology (See Box 2.1).

Components of the examination should include:
- A full medical and developmental history, including a review of past and present treatment and medication;
- A comprehensive physical examination that looks for major physical disorders. It is also important to attend to other characteristics such as skin lesions or physical anomalies that may indicate an etiology of an ID that has not previously been recognized and may impact on presenting behaviors and other symptoms of mental disorders;

- Neurological examination for focal signs (abnormalities such as decreased sensory or motor functions) and "soft" neurological signs (clumsiness, unusual movements);
- Laboratory and biomedical investigation as warranted by findings from above assessments and incorporating knowledge of the biomedical factors that can impact those with mental disorders and ID. Extensive study (e.g., numerous neurobiological investigations such as MRIs or CT scans of the head) is not usually needed, but careful clinical and physical examination and screening for common disorders are warranted. Initial findings may indicate a need for more comprehensive study, and
- Further specialist evaluation (e.g., neurology, genetics, internal medicine, audiology, endocrinology), if indicated by findings from above.

Note that the identification and treatment of substance abuse in individuals with ID is virtually uninvestigated in the research literature despite awareness that this can be a significant problem particularly among individuals with mild ID in relatively independent living settings. This should be considered in the evaluation of biological factors impacting on the clinical presentation.

OBSERVATIONAL ASSESSMENTS

Mental State

The usual format for examining mental state would consist of assessment of appearance, behavior, speech, emotional state, thought, cognition, insight and judgment by direct interview of the client. This has to be adapted to the developmental and functional level of the individual. The assessor must be able to provide more time and flexibility than may be typical practice for other clients without ID. For individuals with mild ID, a formal interview with careful attention to the level of communication is often feasible. With more cognitively limited and nonverbal persons, the assessment may have to take place in different settings (e.g., home, school or day program) and utilize the highly developed observational skills of the clinician. More information may be obtained by interaction between the interviewer and referred individual during an activity; this can help develop a relationship that will allow easier exploration of emotional issues.

The ability to identify internal emotional issues and potentially pathological thought content and patterns should not be underestimated. Careful interview with verbal individuals, after establishing rapport, can lead to identification of symptoms of abnormal mood states (e.g., depression or euphoria), anxiety or fears, obsessive/compulsive disorder as well as delusions, hallucinations, thought disorder and suicidal or aggressive thoughts. Atypical speech patterns such as echolalia, perseveration, unusual voice inflexion or modulation and atypical use of speech in a social context could indicate that a comorbid condition (particularly a Pervasive Developmental Disorder, such as Autism) is present and should be factored into the assessment. At the same time, careful observation of nonverbal behavior can be very informative in all individuals, and observed characteristics are an important component of the assessment of mental state. These include eliciting signs of abnormal activity level (high or low), agitation, atypical movements (e.g., tics, stereotypies, mannerisms), repetitiveness and unusual reactivity to the environment as well as assessing level of alertness, awareness of surroundings, efforts to engage with others and nonverbal communication through gesture and facial expression.

Behavioral Analysis

Persons with ID may be highly sensitive to their environments and much of their behavior may be under the control of situational, environmental stimuli. Reactions to relatively minor events may seem extreme and could reflect a number of factors such as hypersensitivities to noise or social settings, confusion regarding environmental events or inability to express distress through more typical verbal exchange. Given the potential for such situation-specific reactivity and the potential for misinterpretation of observed behavior as due to mental disorder, it is crucial that the evaluating team is able to review patterns of behavior over multiple settings. Ideally, someone from the clinical team should visit the client's residence, school or workplace, noting such things as physical barriers, social interactions with other clients and interactions between the client and his or her family or other caregivers. The goal of this assessment is to identify important individual personal characteristics and responses to social interaction that may be impacting on the presentation of problem behavior disturbances.

In addition, a qualified behavioral psychologist should undertake a functional behavioral analysis (see Chapter 8). The analysis will document the stimuli controlling the client's behavior and estimate the nature and potential success of a subsequent behavioral intervention.

Assessment of the Care-giving System

In assessing the social and environmental factors in a client's life, it is important to recognize the impact the caregivers have on the individual. An understanding of the ways all the various caregivers interact with the client may shed light on the client's current behaviors and functions thereof. What the caregivers say and how they say it has a significant impact upon the client's function, expression of symptoms and emotional well-being. It is well known that for individuals with schizophrenia, being in environments where there is a significant expression of criticism, hostility or intense emotional over-involvement leads to a poorer outcome (Rosenfarb, Nuechterlein, Goldstein, & Subotnik, 2000). The ways the caregivers interact, both within a given setting and from setting to setting, e.g., between residential staff and family of origin or between day program staff and residential staff, is also important. Significant disagreements among caregivers can be confusing to the client and could lead to disruptive or even bizarre behaviors (Nezu et al., 1992).

THE FORMULATION

The formulation is a succinct written appraisal of the important, diagnostically relevant features of the presentation of the individual (history, assessment of mental state, physical assessments, functional abilities and behavioral, social and environmental factors) and how they lead those doing the assessment to the diagnoses. With so many, sometimes contradictory sources of information, it is important to organize and prioritize the data to make the correct multi-axial diagnoses. This formulation guides the treatment planning process and helps determine what needs attention first. For example, the accurate diagnosis of an anxiety disorder may suggest that the prescribing of anti-anxiety medication is indicated. However, the overall assessment may have identified important environmental issues that must be urgently addressed. If not resolved, the anxiety disorder is unlikely to respond to any medication. Alternately, it is inappropriate to delay introduction of appropriate pharmacotherapy for major mental disorders such as bipolar affective disorder or schizophrenia, even if psychosocial issues that could be exacerbating the presenting problems are present.

In developing the formulation, the astute clinician will incorporate the knowledge obtained from the many professional disciplines involved to create order from the assessment findings. The working clinical team can then proceed to appropriately address the identified problem areas and clinical disorders. At times, the diagnosis is not certain and must be given as a hypothesis. Though the assessment is ongoing, appropriate treatment trials may be instituted. In this situation, the multi-axial diagnoses provide a crucial structure for monitoring and assessing treatment priorities and response while allowing longitudinal assessment to clarify the most valid interpretation of the client's presentation.

SUMMARY

In working with individuals who have a combination of a mental disorder and ID, the assessment constitutes the most crucial component of practice. A cursory assessment can lead to either an inaccurate diagnosis or an inadequate appreciation of all of the issues that relate to the presentation of a mental disorder. The wrong diagnosis or a missing component of an evaluation is likely to have long-term consequences such as inappropriate treatment with psychotropic agents. Psychosocial factors of importance may not be addressed, if either not recognized or not factored into the diagnostic assessment. This chapter has provided the rationale for and a description of the structure of a biopsychosocial assessment that should be the standard of evaluation for individuals with mental disorders and ID.

REFERENCES

Aman, M. G., & Singh, N. N. (1986). *Manual: Aberrant behavior checklist*. East Aurora, NY: Slosson Educational Publication.

Aman, M. G., & Singh, N. N. (1994). *Aberrant behavior checklist community supplementary manual*. East Aurora, NY: Slosson Educational Publications.

Ammerman, R. T., Hersen, M., VanHasselt, V. B., Lubetsky, M. J., & Sieck, W. R. (1994). Maltreatment in psychiatrically hospitalized children and adolescents with developmental disabilities: Prevalence and correlates. *Journal of the American Academy of Child and Adolescent Psychiatry, 33*, 567-576.

American Psychiatric Association (2000). *Diagnostic and statistical manual of mental disorders* (Rev., 4th ed.). Washington, DC: American Psychiatric Association.

Burt, D. B., Loveland, K. M., & Lewis, K. R. (1992). Depression and the onset of dementia in adults with Intellectual Disabilities. *American Journal of Intellectual Disabilities, 96*, 502-511.

DiLavore, P. C., Lord, C., & Rutter, M. (1999). The pre-linguistic autism diagnostic observation schedule. *Journal of Autism and Developmental Disorders, 25*, 355-379.

Einfeld, S. L., & Tonge, B. J. (1999). Observations on the use of the ICD-10 guide for Intellectual Disabilities. *Journal of Intellectual Disability Research, 43*, 408-412.

Einfeld, S. J. & Tonge, B. J., (1994). *Manual for the developmental behavior checklist* (Primary Care Version). Victoria, Australia: University of New South Wales and Monash Universities Press.

Engel, G. L. (1977). The need for a new medical model: A challenge for biomedicine. *Science, 196*, 129-136.

Gardner, W. I., & Sovner, R. (1994). *Self-Injurious behaviors: Diagnosis and treatment: A multimodal functional approach*. Philadelphia: VIDA Publishing.

Gardner, W. I., & Whalen, J. P. (1996). A multimodal behavior analytic model for evaluating the effects of medical problems on non-specific behavioral symptoms in persons with developmental disabilities. *Behavioral Interventions, 11*, 147-161.

Haaven, J., Little, R., & Petre-Miller, D. (1990). *Treating intellectually disabled sex offenders: A model residential program*. Orwell, VT: Safer Society Press.

Hurley, A. D. (2001). Axis IV and V: Assessment of persons with Intellectual Disabilities and Developmental Disabilities. *Mental Health Aspects of Developmental Disabilities, 4*, 17-20.

Krug, D. A., Arick, J., & Almond, P. (1980). Behavior checklist for identifying severely handicapped individuals with high levels of autistic behavior. *Journal of Child Psychology and Psychiatry, 21*, 221-229.

Levitas, A., & Gilson S. F. (2001). Predictable developmental crises in the lives of people with Intellectual Disabilities. *Mental Health Aspects of Developmental Disabilities, 4*, 89-100.

Lord, C., Rutter, M., & LeCouter, A. (1994). Autism diagnostic interview-revised: A revised version of a diagnostic interview for caregiver of individuals with possible pervasive development. *Journal of Autism and Developmental Disorders, 24*, 659-685.

Matson J. L. (1997). *The PIIDA manual* (2nd Ed.). Worthington, OH: IDS Publishing Corporation.

Matson, J. L., Gardner, W. I., Coe, D. A., & Sovner, R. (1991) A scale for evaluating emotional disorders in severely and profoundly mentally retarded persons: Development of the Diagnostic Assessment for the Severely Handicapped (DASH) Scale. *British Journal of Psychiatry, 159*, 404-409.

Matson, J. L., Coe, A., Gardner, W. I., & Sovner, R. (1991). A factor analytic study of the diagnostic assessment for the severely handicapped scale. *The Journal of Nervous and Mental Disease, 179*, 553-557.

Meadows, G., Turner, T., Campbell, L., Lewis, S. W., Reveley, M. A., & Murray, R. M. (1991). Assessing schizophrenia in adults with Intellectual Disabilities: A comparative study. *British Journal of Psychiatry, 158*, 103-105.

Moss, S. C. (2001). *The MINI PAS-ADD: An assessment schedule for the detection of mental health problems in adults with learning disability (Intellectual Disabilities)*. Brighton, England: Pavilion Publishing.

Moss, S. C., Patel, P., Prosser, H., Goldberg, D., Simpson, N., Rowe, S., & Luccino, R., (1993). Psychiatric morbidity in older people with moderate and severe learning disability (Intellectual Disabilities). Part 1. Development and reliability of the client interview (The PAS-ADD). *British Journal of Psychiatry, 163*, 471-480.

Moss, S. C., Prosser, H., Costello, H., Simpson, N., Patel, P., Rowe, S., et al. (1998). Reliability and validity of the PAS-ADD checklist for detecting mental disorders in adults with Intellectual Disability. *Journal of Intellectual Disability Research, 42*, 173-183.

Nezu, C. M., Nezu, A. M., & Gill-Weiss, M. J. (1992). *Psychopathology in persons with Intellectual Disabilities: Clinical guidelines for assessment and treatment.* Champaign, IL: Research Press Company.

Nihira, K., Leland, H., & Lambert, N. (1993). *Adaptive behavior scale: Residential and community.* Washington, DC: AAID.

Reiss, S., & Valenti-Hein, D. (1994). Development of a psychopathology rating scale for children with Intellectual Disabilities. *Journal of Consulting and Clinical Psychology, 62*, 28-33.

Reiss, S. (1988). *Test manual for the Reiss Screen for maladaptive behavior.* Worthington, OH: IDS Publishing Corporation.

Rosenfarb, I. S., Nuechterlein, K. H., Goldstein, M. J., & Subotnik, K. L. (2000). Neurocognitive vulnerability, interpersonal criticism, and the emergence of unusual thinking by schizophrenic patients during family transactions. *Archives of General Psychiatry, 57*, 1174-1179.

Ryan, R., & Sunada, K. (1997). Medical evaluations of persons with Intellectual Disabilities referred for psychiatric evaluation. *General Hospital Psychiatry, 19*, 274-280.

Schopler, E., Reichler, R. J., & Renner, B. R. (1988), *The Childhood Autism Rating Scale* (CARS). Los Angeles: Western Psychological Services.

Sovner, R., and Hurley, A. D., (1989). *Psychiatric aspects of mental retardation* Vol. 6: *Reviews.* Washington, DC: AAID.

Sovner, R., & Hurley, A. D. (1999). Facts and fiction concerning Mental Disorders in people with Intellectual Disabilities and Developmental Disabilities. In N. A. Wiesler & R. H. Hanson (Eds.), *Behavior disorder of persons with mental health disorders and severe Developmental Disabilities.* Washington, DC: AAID.

Strohmer, D. C., & Prout, H. T. (1991). *The emotional problems scales.* Odessa, FL: Psychological Assessment Resources.

Turk, V., & Brown, H. (1994). The sexual abuse of adults with learning disability: Results of a two-year incidence survey. *Mental Handicap Research, 6*, 193-216.

WHO (1992). *The international classification of diseases and related health problems.* (10th Ed.). Geneva, Switzerland: World Health Organization.

WHO (1996). *ICD-10 Guide for Intellectual Disabilities.* Geneva, Switzerland: World Health Organization.

3

Mental Disorders in Adults with Intellectual Disability

Howard B. Demb

INTRODUCTION

Current approaches to the diagnosis of mental disorders in persons with intellectual disabilities (ID) include a developmental perspective (Charlot, 1998). This approach to psychopathology presupposes an inherent relationship between developmental level and coping effectiveness (Charlot, 1997). At earlier developmental levels, functioning tends to be reactive, stimulus-bound and driven by external stimuli as well as internal need states. During the course of development the individual becomes increasingly able to plan, control and respond preferentially to either internal stimuli or external forces. Gratification can be delayed and the individual can be more flexible and adaptive.

Population surveys have revealed that people of all ages with ID are more vulnerable to psychopathology than those without ID, and that the prevalence of mental disorders increases as the intellectual level decreases (Dosen & Gielen, 1993; Deb, Matthews, Holt, & Bouras, 2001). There have been a number of hypothesized explanations for these findings. Individuals with ID may have diminished social competence and difficulties coping in a complex environment. Limited adaptive skills may result in the experiencing of fear, a lack of the ability to control stressful events and a sense of uncertainty and insecurity. It is likely that there are a combination of biological, social and environmental factors that interact with cognitive and adaptive behavior deficits to make persons with ID vulnerable, not only to classic mental disorders, but also to the demonstration of behavior disturbances such as excitability, explosiveness, hyperactivity, agitation, irritability, aggression to self and others and destructive and stereotyped behaviors (Ryan, 1996[a]). These behaviors may reflect mental disorders such as mood, anxiety or psychotic disorders; relate to histories of abuse or neglect; be the result of a developmental level far below the chronological age, or relate to the presence of a seizure disorder.

This chapter will present information as to how several standard diagnoses of mental disorders are manifested in adults with ID. The symptoms often present in more subtle ways due to the more simplistic, concrete thinking present in individuals with ID.

SCHIZOPHRENIA AND OTHER PSYCHOTIC DISORDERS

The Diagnostic and Statistical Manual of Mental Disorders - Fourth Edition, Text Revision (DSM-IV-TR, APA 2000) criteria for schizophrenia requires the presence of two or more of the following symptoms:
- Auditory or visual hallucinations;
- Delusions;
- Disorganized speech;
- Grossly disorganized or catatonic behavior, or
- Any of a number of negative symptoms such as the lack of ability to initiate work or self-care, speech that does not provide much information or is irrelevant and flat affect.

Only one symptom is necessary if the delusions are bizarre: if the hallucination is of a voice keeping up a running commentary on the person or if there are two or more voices conversing with each other. These symptoms must have been present for six months and there must be significantly decreased social or occupational functioning. (See DSM-IV-TR for more details.)

It is often hard to discern these symptoms in individuals with ID, especially if they are nonverbal. However, observations of the individual's behavior may suggest that a mental disorder is present (Ryan, 1996[b]). For example, hallucinations may manifest themselves in such ways as:
- Talking or muttering to oneself or appearing to be carrying on a conversation;
- Looking up at the corner of the room and ceiling;
- Nodding as though involved in a conversation;
- Shadowboxing or striking out for no discernible reason;
- Looking over one's shoulder or appearing frightened;
- Staring or appearing preoccupied (possibly caused by a preoccupation with the hallucination);
- Repeatedly brushing unseen material off of the body;
- Grimacing or wincing as though smelling or tasting something foul when one is not eating, or
- Covering the eyes or ears in a quiet room (Weisblatt, 1994).

Delusions can present as:
- Thinking a TV hero is real and a part of one's life;
- Thinking that people are talking about him or her;
- Stating that, or, behaving as if, the food is poisoned;
- Believing someone is trying to hurt him or her;
- Glaring with an intensely angry facial expression at strangers or at individuals who one previously liked, or
- Inspecting or refusing food in a manner suggesting fear.

Disorganized speech may be identified when phrases are disconnected or statements are irrelevant. Other indicators are incoherence, frequent divergence from the topic, echolalia (the apparently senseless repetition of a word or phrase either just spoken by another person or spoken by another person in the past), perseveration (the constant repetition of a meaningless word or phase or the repetition of a behavior or response that may have been appropriate initially but is no longer appropriate), thought blocking (beginning a sentence and then stopping in mid-thought) or lack of reciprocal speech.

Grossly disorganized behavior includes such things as eating from the garbage, urinating in inappropriate places, eating inedibles (when past abilities suggest the individual would know better), drinking out of the toilet or wearing multiple layers of clothing when not warranted by the weather.

Catatonia may be present and is usually seen as a sustained, fixed posture during which time the individual seems to be in a stupor.

Negative symptoms include avolition (an inability to begin or continue in goal-directed self-care, work or social activities), alogia or poverty of speech (a decreased fluency and productivity of speech with brief empty responses to questions, suggesting a diminution of thoughts) and a flattening of affect (the persons face appears immobile and unresponsive, often with a lack of eye contact).

If these symptoms have been present for one month, but less than six, it is called schizophreniform disorder. If all of the symptoms for schizophrenia were present as well as those for a mood disorder (as described in the next section), the diagnosis would be schizoaffective disorder.

Generally, an individual presents the information about delusions and hallucinations verbally. As a result schizophrenia can be diagnosed in the usual manner in a person with fairly good language skills and only mild ID but is more difficult to diagnose in the presence of limited language skills and more severe ID. In this situation observations by others become important factors in making this diagnosis. Parents and staff can assess to what extent the adult's behaviors represent a deterioration or significant change from a previous level of functioning or are in keeping with the adult's developmental level as in uncomplicated ID.

Other signs of schizophrenia include "gating deficits," that is, becoming disorganized because of the onset of an inability to adapt to ordinary sensory stimuli such as the brightness of florescent lights, the noise of an electric heater or conversation outside of the room. This may also occur due to an inability to sort out olfactory, tactile, visual or gustatory sensations (Sovner & Pary, 1993). In this case the disorganization has to do with previously acquired skills, for example, dressing, maintaining hygiene, preparing meals that are lost by the adult or displays of inappropriate sexual behavior (e.g. public masturbation) or unexplained agitation (e.g., swearing or shouting). "Gating deficits" can also be seen in pervasive developmental disorders, for example, autism, in the form of hypersensitivity to local noises or noises of a certain pitch. In the case of pervasive developmental disorder, social skills deficits, inappropriate communication skills and repetitive self-stimulating, behaviors are usually not accompanied by hallucinations or delusions.

The combination of the previously mentioned bizarre behaviors, "gating deficits" and difficulty initiating activities (in the absence of signs or symptoms of a mood disorder) should lead the clinician to consider the diagnosis of schizophrenia. If uncertain that the individual satisfies DSM-IV-TR criteria for schizophrenia, but there is a strong suggestion of the presence of psychosis (without prominent mood symptoms), then the diagnosis of a psychotic disorder not otherwise specified (NOS) should be considered.

Example: Psychosis

P. is a 22-year-old man who has a mild ID. He currently lives in a group home with six other young men. He moved there three months ago. He had previously lived with his mother. Their relationship was very volatile, and they were experiencing great difficulties in living in the same house. He now sees his mother every two weeks in a neutral location.

P. is described as usually being a sociable and polite person who likes to meet new people. However, the group home staff are concerned that for the past month he has not been socializing with the other residents as much as he used to and has been rude to people. He has stopped seeing his girlfriend, saying that she is nosy and always asking him questions. His appearance is also not what it used to be; he wears the same clothes for days on end, and the staff cannot remember the last time that he bathed.

An urgent assessment is requested when he withdraws further. At that time his speech is incoherent, and he is unable to answer questions. Each time someone tries to make eye contact with him, he hides his face with his hands in a child-like manner. He is unkempt and wears no shoes. He curls up into a ball shape and giggles and mumbles, seemingly to himself.

P. was admitted to a local psychiatric hospital inpatient unit. He was treated with an antipsychotic medication and was discharged back to his group home in three weeks. At discharge, his speech was coherent; he was able to care for himself; his affect was appropriate, and he engaged with other people. There was no evidence of hallucinations. P. was to continue to take his antipsychotic medication and was to be followed as an outpatient by the mental health clinic of an agency that serves adults with ID.

MOOD DISORDERS

The major mood disorders include: dysthymia (a chronic state of mild to moderate depression that has been present for two years); major depressive disorder (severe sadness, loss of interest in formerly pleasurable activities and disturbances in sleep, appetite, energy level and activity level lasting two weeks or longer), and bipolar disorders (serious depression alternating with manic or hypomanic episodes of varying lengths and frequencies). Individuals with ID suffer from these disorders with a frequency at least as high as those without ID (Roberts, 1986). In persons with mild ID, the symptoms are similar to those among individuals without ID although they may be expressed in a simpler and more concrete way, for example, reporting feeling sick rather than identifying the emotion of feeling sad. In adults with more severe ID, especially nonverbal adults, there are often few if any verbal complaints. Observable data must be used to determine if a mood disorder is present in such adults. This data includes sleep records, changes in weight (accompanied by changes in food intake associated with a loss of or increased appetite), notations of unexplained sadness, crying, becoming happy and laughing for no apparent reason or the onset of unprovoked aggression.

Behavioral symptoms must be assessed in the context of change over time. In adults, the symptoms may have been present in a chronic or mixed state for many years and thus appear not to cycle. If the caregivers are unfamiliar with the individual's early history and have never seen a change in behavior, the symptoms may be overlooked and never reported to a mental health care provider. Rapid cycling of mood in persons with ID who have bipolar disorders is reported to occur more often than in other populations (Tucker, 2002).

Before making a definitive diagnosis, the effects of medication should be considered as a possible etiology for mood disorders. Agitation associated with motor restlessness (akathisia) that mimics a manic symptom can be a result of an antipsychotic medication. Antidepressants can result in a switch from depression to mania. Benzodiazepines can result in manic-like euphoria (mania or hypomania) or manic-like episodes of disinhibition with aggressive or self-injurious behaviors (Larson et al., 2001; Wilson, Lott, & Tsai, 1998). The use of beta-blockers may increase the risk of depression (Lumley & Miltenberger, 1997).

Depression

Five of the nine behavioral or subjective symptoms listed in DSM-IV-TR (APA 2000) must be present to make the diagnosis of a major depression (fewer for dysthymia or depression not otherwise specified). Any of these symptoms can be observed in a client, regardless of their language capabilities or level of ID (Szymanski, et al., 1998). These symptoms include: (See Table 3.1.)

- Evidence of a depressed mood. Things such as these may manifest this: tearfulness, an increase in somatic complaints or irritability. At times, the examiner must rely on the description by caregivers of a change in the individual from being happy, smiling, laughing or having a sense of humor to an absence of these characteristics.
- A diminished interest or lack of pleasure in activities may be shown by no longer interacting with friends, appearing apathetic about activities enjoyed in the past or refusing to participate in activities or outings.
- A change in appetite may be expressed as refusal to go to the dining table or refusal to eat once there. This may be reported by caregivers only as non-compliance and should be asked about specifically. Food stealing and/or hoarding may also occur. Careful recording of serial weights is important, as this may be the only objective evidence of a change in appetite.
- Insomnia or increased sleeping can occur. Sometimes behavioral disturbances occur at bedtime and mask the difficulty that an individual has falling asleep. It is important to know if an individual is sleeping through the night, awakens early or is sleeping longer than usual. Sleep data that records the number of hours slept is helpful in this assessment.
- Psychomotor agitation or retardation may be present. Agitation may be represented as pacing, the inability to sit still or a general restlessness. Conversely, there may be a complete slowing in motor activities manifested in such ways as walking very slowly, eating slowly or taking a long time to do things.
- Fatigue or loss of energy may be manifested by a decrease in productivity or regression in skills. Individuals may sleep more, stay in bed or refuse to do activities.

Table 3.1
Criteria for Major Depressive Episode*

Symptoms from five or more groups from this list must be present, and one must be a depressed mood or loss of interest in things.

1. Depressed mood
- Tearfulness
- Increased somatic complaints
- Irritability
- Decreased smiling or laughing
- Decreased sense of humor

2. Loss of interest in usual activities
- Stops interacting with friends
- Shows no interest in things
- Seems lazy, bored or indifferent
- Refuses to participate in previously favored activities
- Refuses to participate in anything

3. Weight loss or gain or a change in appetite
- Refuses to eat meals
- Refuses to go to the table
- Refuses to eat with others
- Steals food
- Hoards food

4. Decreased or increased sleep
- Behavior disturbances at bedtime
- Changes in hours of sleep
- Trouble staying in bed
- Spends most of the time in bed

5. Significant agitation (rapid movements) or slow movements
- Paces
- Unable to sit still
- Restlessness
- Increase in self-injury
- Decreased speech
- Trouble completing activities of daily living
- Unable to finish tasks
- Aggression
- Slow in doing tasks
- Runs away
- Increase in stereotypies

6. Tired or low energy almost daily
- Decrease in productivity
- Regression in skills
- Refuses to do as requested

7. Feeling unimportant, worthless or guilty
- States such things as: "Nobody likes me." and "I can't do this job."
- Destroys possessions

8. Difficulty concentrating or making decisions
- Decrease in productivity
- Regression of skills
- Inability to finish a task
- Decreased attention to a task
- Appears to be "non-compliant"
- Says, "I don't know."

9. Talks about death, dying or suicide, including specific plans or an actual suicide attempt
- Deliberately does things that are potentially lethal;
- Begins self-injurious behavior;
- Offers self up to peers who are known to be aggressive, and/or
- Talks about family members who are deceased (Dosen & Gielen, 1993), may talk about joining them.

*Symptoms in bold are DSM-IV-TR criteria paraphrased (See DSM-IV-TR for details.) Beneath them are some of the ways these symptoms may be manifested in an individual with ID.

- Feelings of worthlessness or excessive or inappropriate guilt may be expressed in such statements as "nobody likes me" or "I can't do this job" or by behaviors such as destroying or throwing out possessions.
- Diminished ability to think, concentrate or make decisions may also be expressed by decreased productivity or regression of skills. An individual may begin a task but not follow it through. Decreased attention to the task may also occur. Staff may report that the individual is unable to make a decision, constantly changes his or her mind or is non-compliant.
- Recurrent thoughts of death (not just fear of dying), recurrent suicidal ideation or an actual suicide attempt may occur. This may be expressed verbally; as deliberate, potentially lethal acts; as self-injurious behavior or offering oneself up to peers who are known to be aggressive. Some individuals may talk frequently about family members who are deceased (Dosen & Gielen, 1993).

Individuals with depression and ID may acutely decompensate and show loss of previously acquired skills (e.g., poor school or day-program performance). Such individuals may appear regressed or agitated at such times (Dana, 1993). Irritability, anger and aggression (including self-injurious behaviors) are often a feature of an affective disturbance, and adults with depression and ID are more likely to display overt aggression than are individuals with depressed average cognitive abilities (Charlot, 1998).

Example: Depression

T. is a 32-year-old woman who has severe ID and autism. She lives in a supported house with three other people and 24-hour staff support. She has no speech and uses no signs. She makes her basic needs known by holding a staff member's hand and leading him or her to whatever she wants.

A referral to mental health services was precipitated when she recently started to scream, especially in the mornings. On two occasions another resident hit her when she was screaming.

Staff had noticed that her mood was a lot worse in the mornings. She became agitated and screamed when staff tried to support her to get dressed. She sometimes threw herself on the floor and hit herself. Also, on some occasions she pulled at her hair, and there were now bald patches on the sides of her head. The staff felt her mood improved as the day went on. She refused her breakfast on most mornings but ate lunch and dinner, although not to the extent that she used to. She had been seen crying in her bedroom without any apparent cause. Previously she had enjoyed a wide range of activities at home and in the community; now she appeared withdrawn and worried.

T. was started on an antidepressant. Five weeks after she was administered a therapeutic dose, her symptoms began to improve. She was no longer irritable in the morning; she stopped crying, and she was less withdrawn. She also began to engage in activities that she had previously enjoyed. The plan was to keep T. on the antidepressant for six months, and then to gradually decrease the antidepressant dosage and monitor her response to determine whether she still needed it.

Mania

A manic episode is a distinct period of abnormally and persistently elevated, expansive or irritable mood that lasts for at least one week (or less if the person is hospitalized because of symptoms of the manic episode) (DSM-IV-TR, 2000). In individuals with ID these mood states may be expressed in ways that are less clearly identifiable (Lowry 1998; Szymanski et al., 1998). They include shouting, yelling, screaming, silliness, excessive smiling or laughing, dressing or wearing make-up in an exaggerated fashion, teasing, singing and dancing (sometimes with people they don't know or never liked). These behaviors may be labeled "manipulative" rather than recognized as evidence of elevated or expansive mood. Irritability can often be identified readily in someone with ID. It should also be considered when observing such things as an angry face, grumpy or grouchiness, being extremely upset with others, aggression, spitting at others or striking out at a previously liked person. Seghorn & Ball (2000) suggest that these symptoms often manifest themselves in behaviors that may be confused with mannerisms and actions seen in persons with ID, masking the diagnosis.

To make the manic diagnosis there must also be symptoms and behaviors from three of the seven non-mood categories listed below. If the mood symptom is just irritability there must be symptoms and behaviors from four categories. The categories and examples of some of the ways that they may manifest in individuals with ID are as follows: (See Table 3.2.)

Inflated Self-Esteem or Grandiosity

Behaviors that suggest inflated self-esteem or grandiosity include unrealistic goals, perhaps related to a belief that they do not have ID. Some may even state that they are not disabled. Inflated self-esteem may be hard to identify and easy to overlook. It may be expressed by comments like "I can do that," when it is an activity that they cannot perform, by bossing others around or refusing to do what others ask of them, such as expected chores. Grandiosity in a person with ID is usually not as exaggerated as in someone without ID but can include such claims as having a relationship with a famous person.

Decreased Need for Sleep

Such adults may feel rested after only three hours of sleep. Note should be taken if an individual is up all or much of the night, displays a great deal of energy and does not attempt to nap throughout the day. Expressing the lack of need for sleep may also occur through an increase in maladaptive behavior at night, especially if the person's mood is irritable.

More Talkative Than Usual or Pressure To Keep Talking

Non-stop talking or constant vocalization may be the way pressured speech presents. Someone who likes humor may increase the number of jokes that they tell. There can be an increase in the intensity of whatever means a person uses to communicate. Some adults with severe ID communicate distress by head banging, which may increase during mania. Other adults with less severe ID may use signing or gesturing to communicate, behaviors that may also increase during mania.

Flights of Ideas or Subjective Experience So That Thoughts Are Racing

Rapid shifts in conversation from one topic to another should alert the observer to this symptom. An attempt to work on several projects at one time or jumping from one to another without finishing anything may reflect racing thoughts. Non-stop talking may also be a sign of this symptom. This can be tested, in part, by seeing if the individual can stop the behavior for an extended time, when requested to do so.

Distractibility

Distractibility involves attention that is too easily drawn to unimportant or irrelevant external stimuli. This may be readily observed if the individual constantly turns to see where a new noise is coming from or repeatedly looking at what others are doing rather than staying focused on their own activity. A decrease in productivity at work or school could also be a result of this. Some individuals are described as "getting into everyone's business," which should alert the observer to look for additional signs of distractibility symptoms from other categories such as inflated self-esteem or grandiosity.

Increase in Goal-Directed Activity or Psychomotor Agitation

Any increase in activity (socially or sexually, at work or school) should suggest the possibility of this symptom group. This could run the gamut from starting lots of projects (though often not completing them) to pacing constantly and rarely sitting down. Other behaviors may include increased dancing or singing, intrusiveness, aggression, assault, disruption, increase in masturbation or the presence of sexual behaviors in public. For individuals who are functioning in the severe and profound range of ID, this symptom may manifest by doing more of what they already do such as ripping clothing, eating rapidly, eating more, exhibiting self-stimulatory behavior and a change in frequency or intensity of rituals.

Excessive Involvement in Pleasurable Activities That Have a High Potential for Painful Consequences

Since most adults with ID are on a fixed budget this symptom should be considered when the adult engages in unrestrained spending sprees such as spends all of their week's allotment in the first day or steals. There may also be an increase in sexual activity that may include increased masturbation, public displays of suggestively sexual behavior or touching, hugging or grabbing strangers.

The additional criteria for making the mania diagnosis is that the mood disturbance causes at least one of the following:
- Marked impairment in day program, work or interpersonal relationships;
- Need for hospitalization to protect from harming self or others, or
- Psychotic features such as hallucinations or delusions.

Example: Mania

D. is a 34-year-old man with mild ID. At age 17 he stopped doing most of his usual activities, became irritable when asked to do chores and began pacing. He was admitted

Table 3.2
Criteria for Manic Episode

A. An individual must have a mood that is elevated, more expansive or irritable Shouting, yelling, screaming Bossing Refusal to do what others ask, such as expected chores Aggression or property destruction Silliness Dressing or making up in an exaggerated fashion Teasing Singing Dancing with people without a previous relationship Striking out at or rejecting a previously liked person
B. While the mood is elevated or irritable there must be symptoms from three or more of the following groups (four symptoms if the mood is only irritable):
1. Evidence that the individual has grandiose ideas or a higher self-esteem than is realistic Unrealistic goals Belief that they do not have mental retardation Belief that they can do a job though they have no such skills Bosses others around Claims to have a relationship with a famous person
2. Sleeps fewer hours at night but feels well-rested Up all or much of the night Displays a great deal of energy and doesn't attempt to nap throughout the day Increase in maladaptive behavior at night.
3. Rapid, pressured speech or talks more than usual Non-stop talking or constant vocalization Any increase in intensity of whatever means a person uses to communicate (e.g., head banging) Increase in joking
4. Sense that thoughts are racing or rushing from one idea to another Rapid shifts in conversation from one topic to another A high activity level Rushing from one thing to another Attempts to work on several projects at one time
5. Inability to ignore distractions in the environment Distractibility Inability to pay attention to a task Loss of productivity at work or at school
6. Increase in appropriate activities or agitation Intrusiveness such as touching people, going into others' rooms or interfering with someone else's activities Public masturbation Notable increase in masturbation Aggression, assault, disruption Increased eating Self-stimulatory behavior Change in frequency or intensity of rituals
7. Engaging in behaviors that may be risky or lead to negative consequences but bring pleasure in the moment Increased sexual preoccupation Increased sexual activity Increased or frequent masturbation Overeating Hoarding Stealing things to keep or give away

*Symptoms in bold are DSM-IV-TR criteria, paraphrased (See DSM-IV-TR for details.) Beneath them are some of the ways these symptoms may be manifested in an individual with ID.

to the hospital where he was observed talking to himself, giggling inappropriately and constantly touching other people. He was described as "attention-seeking." His demeanor was very childlike. He was begun on psychotropic medication. After one year these were stopped, and he soon became symptomatic. He began yelling and swearing in a very loud voice, talked rapidly, became very aggressive, would not do anything anyone else asked him to do and began talking about Power Rangers talking to him and scaring him. At times he was observed talking back or waving his hands in the air. He was begun on an antipsychotic and a mood stabilizer and has done very well.

Hypomania

Hypomania is similar to mania, but need only be present for four days, has no psychotic features and does not require hospitalization. The mood symptoms may, or may not, cause significant impairment in social, occupational or other important areas of functioning.

Example: Hypomania

J. is a 22-year-old single woman with mild ID. She lives with her parents and attends a day habilitation program. For several months staff have been noticing that she has been laughing and grinning a lot, turning cartwheels on break, and rushing to do her work, but, because she is so easily distracted, she is unable to finish tasks that she used to do readily. Her parents report that she has been up in the middle of the night and awakens them, sometimes from the sounds of moving her bedroom furniture around, other times by showering. Often they would find her dressed for program at 3 o'clock in the morning, never needing a nap nor appearing to be tired during the rest of the day. She was referred for assessment because she was becoming quite irritable, yelling and swearing, which was very unlike her, and saying that she didn't need anyone to tell her what to do. When she was seen for assessment, she talked non-stop. The mental health team was not able to complete the interview because she could not be interrupted. She responded to treatment with lithium and was her usual self within two weeks.

ANXIETY DISORDERS

Anxiety is a frequent symptom in adults with or without ID, and anxiety disorders are often comorbid with many other mental disorders. Anxiety, with or without comorbid depression, is a frequent referral complaint among persons with mild ID (Barnhill & Horrigan, 2002).

Adults with ID and poor verbal skills may have difficulty communicating their distress regarding symptoms of anxiety. If the distress results in non-compliance, aggression, screaming or other maladaptive behaviors, the anxiety disorder may go unrecognized. Anxiety disorders in persons with ID are typically under-recognized because of the accompanying intensity of disruptive behaviors. A broad range of anxiety disorders have been reported in persons with ID, including generalized anxiety disorder, panic disorders, posttraumatic stress disorder (PTSD), obsessive-compulsive disorder (OCD) and phobias. These include both specific phobias (an intense fear of, and avoidance of, specific objects or situations e.g., fear of dogs or fear of lightning) and social phobias (an intense fear of being humiliated) (Turk & Brown, 1994). Psychosocial stress factors, including fragile self-esteem, fear of failing, or loss of caregivers, may contribute to anxiety disorders. When trying to describe feeling anxious, people with ID are likely to use terms such as "nervousness" or "shakiness". Upon questioning, some anxious individuals can describe physical symptoms of anxiety such as tightness in the chest, heart pounding, sweating or tension in the muscles. For persons who do not use spoken language to communicate, the observer must recognize physical signs of anxiety. These may include an excessively upright rigid posture, tense jaw muscles, excessive perspiration, rapid breathing, flushing, chewing fingernails (or toenails), mild tics that do not meet criteria for a separate tic disorder, grinding teeth or some sort of self-abusive behavior.

Obsessive-Compulsive Disorder (OCD)

An obsessive-compulsive disorder (OCD) consists of recurrent distressing thoughts (obsessions) that produce anxiety or uncontrollable repetitive behaviors (compulsions) that are intended to reduce anxiety. Their occurrence must cause severe distress or be so time consuming that they cause significant impairment in functioning (DSM-IV-TR, 2000). The obsessions may take the form of repetitive words, thoughts, fears, memories, numbers, pictures or dramatic scenes. The compulsions may take the form of hand-washing, hair pulling, ordering, checking and rechecking or mental acts like counting, praying or repeating words silently. These symptoms last more than one hour each day and cause significant distress or interfere with normal functioning.

Repetitive behaviors in nonverbal individuals with ID may be difficult to categorize. The distinctions among self-stimulatory or stereotypic behaviors and those that result from compulsions are difficult to discern when they are carried out by persons who cannot describe obsessional thoughts or identify felt anxiety, when blocked from performing a compulsive behavior. Repetitive behaviors such as hoarding objects, flicking lights on and off, tidying and rearranging have all been considered suggestive of the diagnosis of an OCD in an individual with ID (American Academy of Child and Adolescent Psychiatry, 1999). Even some forms of self- injurious behavior (SIB), especially when accompanied by self-restraint, suggest ego-dystonic symptoms (a behavior in which the adult does not wish to engage), suggestive of an OCD.

Posttraumatic Stress Disorder (PTSD)

The symptoms associated with PTSD include things like avoidance of people or places that might arouse recollections of the trauma, intrusive flashbacks or re-experiencing of the traumatic event (e.g., abuse), a restricted range of affect or a sense of a foreshortened future (e.g., not expecting to have a normal life span). Children and adults with ID are more vulnerable to abuse than persons without ID because of significant dependency upon caregivers, a tendency to want to please others and a lack of understanding of their rights. Some aggressive behaviors in persons with severe to profound ID may represent manifestations of PTSD in which the vulnerable individual responds aggressively to situations reminiscent of earlier abuse or severe stress. Behavior that might appear to indicate psychosis (e.g., brushing unseen objects or material off of the body, acting in an aggressive way when nobody is around or being fearful, anxious and cowering when there is no observable danger) may reflect a re-experiencing (flashback) or a re-enacting (acting as if the traumatic event were recurring) phenomenon as part of a PTSD. Flashbacks in a

Table 3.3
Tics

Type	Examples
Simple Motor Tics	
Chronic motor tics (brief jerking movements)	Blinking Nose twitching Head jerking Limb jerking
Dystonic motor tics (slow, a briefly sustained abnormal posture)	Sustained eye closure (blepharospasm) Ocular deviations Tooth grinding (bruxism) Mouth opening Neck twisting (torticollis) Shoulder rotation
Tonic tics (an isometric contraction)	Tensing abdominal muscles Tensing limb muscles
Complex Motor Tics	Head shaking Trunk bending or gyrating Brushing hair Touching, throwing, hitting, jumping, kicking Making rude gestures Grabbing one's genitalia or making other lewd or obscene gestures (copropraxia) Imitating others' gestures (echopraxia) Burping Vomiting, retching
Simple Phonic Tics	Sniffing Throat clearing Grunting Squeaking Screaming Coughing Barking Blowing Making sucking sounds

person with ID may be represented by grimacing or wincing as the person re-experiences the traumatic event. Television shows or movies with scenes of aggression may unwittingly trigger these. Wearing multiple layers of clothing may be a symptom of an unconscious desire to try to ward off recurrent abuse.

Tics, Stereotypic Movement Disorders and Self-Injurious Behaviors

Tics are rapid, sudden, intermittent, non-rhythmic, recurrent, involuntary or semi-voluntary movements (motor tics) or sounds (vocal tics) (Jankovic, 1997). Motor tics can be simple (involving only a single muscle group) or complex (involving more than one muscle group). Phonic or vocal tics can also be simple or complex. Examples of motor and phonic tics are listed in Table 3.3.

Motor and phonic tics are often preceded by premonitory sensations that consist of sensations of pricking, tingling or creeping on the skin or other forms of discomfort. The discomforts are often localized, for example, a burning feeling in the eye before an eye blink, nasal stuffiness before a sniff or a sore throat before throat clearing or grunting. These sensations are temporarily relieved after the tic is executed (Jankovic, 2001).

Some complex, repetitive movements and sounds may be considered a compulsion when they are preceded by or associated with a feeling of anxiety or a fear that something bad will happen if they are not promptly and properly executed. Nonverbal individuals have difficulty in communicating these distinctions. Tics are the clinical hallmark of Tourette's syndrome (TS) consisting of multiple motor and vocal tics that do not necessarily occur simultaneously. TS usually begins in childhood and waxes and wanes over time (Freeman et al., 2000). (TS is discussed further in the next chapter). Stereotypic movement disorders are usually more complex than movements seen in Tourette's syndrome. Individuals with mental retardation engage in high rates of stereotypic behaviors that can occur with or without self-injurious behaviors (SIB) (Barnhill & Horrigan, 2002). Stimulatory stereotypies of a non-self-injurious nature are seen in Prader-Willi, Cornelia DeLange and Fragile X syndrome (Gardner & Sovner, 1994).

The DSM-IV-TR introduced the specifier "with self-injurious behavior" (p. 34) to the diagnosis of stereotypic movement disorder for those chronic stereotyped acts that either result in direct physical damage or potentially endanger the physical well-being of the person displaying the behaviors. This diagnosis is indicated if the stereotypic behavior leads to significant functional impairment requiring treatment. SIBs can take the form of:

- Head banging;
- Face and/or head slapping;
- Biting various body parts;
- Cutting or burning the skin;
- Pulling, poking, scratching various body parts, for example, hair pulling, scratching and picking at wounds, eye poking and gouging, pinching, rectal digging and teeth grinding;
- Placing objects in body cavities, for example, ears and nose;
- Aerophogia (excessive or prolonged air swallowing);
- Psychogenic polydypsia (water drinking that greatly exceeds physiologic requirements);
- Rumination (repeated vomiting with the re-ingestion of food), and
- Pica (consumption of non-edible substances, for example, cigarette butts, twigs, feces) (Gardner & Sovner, 1994).

The lower the person's I.Q., the more frequent, severe and treatment resistant the SIBs are likely to be. Other risk factors for SIB include:

- Communication deficits, especially expressive skill deficits;
- Sensory disability, for example, blindness;
- Brain injury;

- Seizure disorders;
- Pervasive developmental disorders;
- Specific medical disorders like Lesch-Nyhan syndrome;
- Histories of lengthy institutional living;
- Borderline personality disorder;
- Various forms of psychosis;
- Major depressive disorder, and
- Medication side effects, for example, akathisia (Gardner & Sovner, 1994).

PICA AND OTHER EATING DISORDERS

Anorexia and bulimia nervosa are relatively rare in the population of individuals with ID in the moderate to severe range, but a disorder known as "pica" is fairly common and, along with rumination (bringing up and re-chewing one's food repeatedly), is seen with greater frequency as the severity of intellectual disability increases. Pica is an eating disorder that is manifested by a craving for oral ingestion of a given substance that is unusual in kind (non-food) and/or quantity (food). DSM-IV-TR gives a more restrictive definition in that it does not include food substances as it states "the essential features of pica is the persistent eating of non-nutritious substance for a period of at least one month." Individuals with all levels of intelligence, of all ages, of both sexes and from a variety of racial and socioeconomic background engage in pica.

The more common forms of pica and the names given to these forms include (Lacey, 1993):
- Pagophagia (ice),
- Geophagia (clay),
- Plumbophagia (lead),
- Amylophagia (starch),
- Coprophagia (feces),
- Cautopyreophagia (burnt matches),
- Tricophagia (hair) and
- Lithophagia (stone).

PERSONALITY DISORDERS

A personality disorder is:
- An enduring pattern of inner experience and behavior;
- A marked deviation from the expectations of the individuals culture;
- Pervasive and inflexible;
- Present from adolescence or early adulthood;
- Stable over time;
- The pattern of behavior leads to distress or impairment, or
- A long-standing pattern of maladaptive behavior.

One must be careful to separate signs of personality disorder from signs of emotional immaturity when observing a person with ID. The most common personality disorders reported in individuals with ID are avoidant, antisocial, paranoid and dependent (Reiss, 1994). Adults with ID can also have a borderline personality disorder. These disorders have the following characteristics:

Avoidant Personality

- Pervasive social inhibition resulting in the avoidance of occupational activities that involve significant interpersonal contact;
- Hypersensitivity to negative evaluation and fears of criticism, disapproval or rejection, and
- Viewing self as socially inept, personally unappealing or inferior to others.

Antisocial Personality

- A pervasive disregard for the rights of others;
- A failure to conform to social norms with regard to lawful behavior;
- Deceitful;
- Irritable and aggressive;
- Impulsivity and disregard to the safety of others;
- Irresponsible;
- Takes advantage of others;
- Care must be taken to ensure that these behaviors exist despite the individual's ability to know better and not as a reflection of inadequate social skills, and
- Characteristics of this personality disorder must be present since the age of 15, but it cannot be diagnosed unless the individual is at least 18 years old (DSM-IV-TR, 2000).

Paranoid Personality

- Being distrustful and suspicious of others;
- Bearing grudges, angry and hostile;
- Being Tense;
- Being Guarded, and
- Feeling misunderstood or victimized.

Dependent Personality

- A need to be taken care of;
- A fear of separation;
- Feeling helpless when alone;
- Clinging, submissive behavior;
- Lets others assume responsibility;
- Unwilling to initiate projects;

- Needs constant advice and reassurance, and
- In an individual with ID, a vulnerability exists to be taken advantage of by others (Dana, 1993; Harvard Mental Health Letter, 2000; Westen & Shedler, 1999).

Borderline Personality

- Unstable relationships with others including stress-related distrust and suspicion of others;
- Marked mood swings;
- Difficulty controlling anger, and
- Impulsivity with the possibility of self-abuse or suicidal gestures.
  (See DSM-IV-TR, 2000 for more specific criteria.)

Example: Personality Disorder

J. is a 25-year-old man who has a mild ID. During his school years he was frequently in trouble at school. His peers easily influenced him, and they would often persuade him to steal things for them, pick on other children and play pranks on the teachers. He was suspended on several occasions. At the age of 9 he was caught in the school art room tearing up everybody's work.

He left school at 16 and got a job in a local supermarket. Shortly afterwards he began a relationship with a girl. After three weeks he asked her to marry him; he had already bought a ring. He became extremely agitated when she said, "No," shouted at her and then hit her across the face several times. The relationship ended, but the girl did not report the incident. Shortly after that he met another girl. After a couple of months he asked her if they could get an apartment together. She said, "No," that it was too early but maybe in the future. He ended the relationship and was verbally abusive in doing so. A few days later his mother found him in his bedroom. He was drunk and had made superficial cuts to his arms. His mother tried to get him to go the hospital, but he refused. She pleaded with him, but he became verbally abusive and threatened to hit her. He was withdrawn and uncommunicative for several weeks afterwards.

A couple of months later, while at work, he began talking to a young female customer. She was not very keen on talking to him and politely tried to finish the conversation. As she walked away, he made abusive comments to her. She immediately reported this to the store manager. The manager reprimanded him and reminded him that there had been previous episodes of quarrelling with staff and customers. J. became angry and physically assaulted his manager. The police were called and J. was arrested. While in the police station cell, J. began to repeatedly bang his head against the wall. A psychiatrist was called to assess him.

The psychiatrist felt that J. had a personality disorder with poor impulse control, difficulty with interpersonal relationships, affective instability, difficulty controlling angry feelings and evidence of self-injurious behaviors. The psychiatrist recommended a low dose of an antipsychotic medication and counseling. J. was released on the condition that he follow through with the above recommendations.

SEXUAL DISORDER

Sexual behavior of individuals with ID is learned, shaped and reinforced by environmental factors. When individuals with ID are functioning within a mainstream environment, their sexual behavior is similar to the sexual behavior of their same-age peers. Conversely, when individuals with ID reside in atypical environments (e.g., institutions) their sexual behavior is correspondingly atypical (e.g., inappropriate masturbation, non-volitional homosexuality) (Edgerton, 1973; Gabhard, 1973). Individuals with ID appear capable of appropriate sexual self-control in a variety of settings (Abraham et al., 1998). Self-control is the product of internal regulation, not external constraints.

However, there is an increased risk of sex offenses in the population of individuals with ID. The majority of sex offenders with ID are youths or young men functioning in the mild to borderline intellectual range. Sex offenders with ID share many features in common with sex offenders that do not have ID. As a group they show a high incidence of adjustment problems at school, delinquency and other behavior problems, including non-sex offenses, mental disorders, organic brain damage, minor physical defects, family psychopathology and psychosocial deprivation. Many have shy, immature personalities, and a significant proportion show sociopathic traits. Sexual naiveté, inability to understand normal sexual relationships, lack of relationship skills, difficulties in mixing with the opposite sex and a low level of pre-offense heterosexual experiences are prominent features in all studies (Day, 1994; Day, 1997).

In addition to these features shared with sex offenders that do not have ID, there are a number of specific psychopathological factors common to sex offenders with ID. These individuals show gross deficiencies in sociosexual knowledge, the law and behavioral codes relating to sexual behavior. They also have gross deficiencies in gender appropriateness and have difficulty distinguishing between deviant and non-deviant behavior. They do not have appropriate ideas of what constitutes a consensual relationship (Murphy, 1983).

There is a high prevalence of victims of abuse among individuals with ID (Lumley & Millenberger, 1997; Turk & Brown, 1994). This can result in posttraumatic stress disorder (Beail & Warden, 1995; Seghorn & Ball, 2000). There is no evidence that the incidence of sexual dysfunction (sexual desire disorders, sexual arousal disorders, orgasmic disorders or sexual pain disorders) is any more frequent in the population of individuals with ID than in the general population.

EPILEPSY AND INTELLECTUAL DISABILITY

Epilepsy is one of the most common disorders associated with ID (Rici, 1993). The frequency and severity of epilepsy varies universally with the level of ID (Roberts, 1986). Epilepsy is associated with an elevated risk of mental disorders (Rutter, 1970). Psychopathology can emerge at any point during the cycle of a seizure among individuals with epilepsy. An individual may begin to suffer from irritability, anxiety, depressed mood and poor concentration or sleep disturbance prior to a seizure (prodrome). These symptoms can be present for several days prior to a seizure and can disappear after a seizure. In some persons, the prodrome can consist of confusional episodes, catatonia (either motoric immobility, excessive apparently purposeless motor activity or extreme negativism e.g., resisting attempts to be moved) or psychosis (So, 1996).

"Post ictally," that is, the period after the seizures, the person can be confused, anxious, disoriented, agitated or have rapid and abrupt shifts in mood (labile). Some individuals have lucid intervals between seizures with intact orientation and memory followed by prolonged periods of mental impairment. This disorder, "interictally," that is, the period between seizures, may have a distinct depressive aspect with irritability, depressed mood, lack of energy, anxiety, sleep disorder and may switch to hypomania, suggesting cycling of a bipolar state (Blumer, 1991). Interictal psychosis may present with atypical clinical features with brief periods of positive symptoms associated with adequate social relatedness and normal affect. Psychosis often appears as seizure frequency declines and often after 10 to 15 years of seizure activity. Factors for long-term risk for psychosis include: onset of seizures in adolescence, difficulty with control and being female (Trimble, 1991).

It is unlikely that there is an epileptic personality. Maladaptive personality profiles have been described that include: hyper-religiosity, hyposexuality, hypergraphia (doing a good deal of writing), irritability, suspiciousness, a preoccupation with philosophical and moral concerns and humorlessness, but large scale studies do not support the idea of a specific personality type associated with seizure disorders (Benson, 1986; Tucker, 2002).

SUMMARY

Since most mental disorders are manifested by essentially the same symptoms in adults with ID as in the general population, a diagnosis of a mental disorder in an adult with ID can usually be made with some confidence. However, since many diagnostic criteria involve an individual's verbal communication, and many symptoms are not specific for a given diagnosis, diagnosing a mental disorder in adults with severe or profound ID and limited or no verbal skills, can be difficult. When adults with ID are not able to describe their feelings or to explain their actions one must use every resource available as a source of information, with emphasis on the observations of caregivers. The clinician should obtain information about not only the adult's symptoms but also significant aspects of the environment, the nature of social interactions and the developmental level. The task then is to see if the symptoms fit into a definable mental disorder. If a nonverbal adult with a severe ID, who has lost a parent, begins to lose interest in taking care of himself, appears sad, cries often and has significant changes in his or her eating, sleeping and energy level, one can be reasonably confident that the adult has a depression. Or, in another instance, sudden loss of interest in personal hygiene in a nonverbal adult with severe ID might be the result of a psychotic disorder, if the adult demonstrates behavior consistent with the presence of hallucinations or delusions as described earlier.

There are times when, despite the best efforts at trying to diagnose a mental disorder, the behavior problems of an adult with severe and profound ID do not fit into any diagnostic scheme. In such cases, it is best to not make a diagnosis but to watch and wait for additional data to clarify the nature of the problem. In the future, contributions from neuroscience, molecular biology and a better understanding of genetic environmental interactions may open up new approaches to the diagnosis of mental disorders in these difficult to diagnose cases.

REFERENCES

Abraham, P. R., Parker, T., & Weisberg, S. R. (1998). Sexual expression of mentally retarded people: Educational and legal implications. *American Journal on Mental Retardation 93*, 328-334.

American Academy of Child and Adolescent Psychiatry (1999). Practice parameters for the assessment and treatment of children, adolescents, and adults with mental retardation and comorbid mental disorders. *Journal of the American Academy of Child and Adolescent Psychiatry, 38*(Suppl.), 5S –31S.

American Psychiatric Association (2000). *Diagnostic and statistical manual of mental disorders* (Rev. 4th ed.).Washington, DC: American Psychiatric Association.

Barnhill, L. J. (1999). Epilepsy, mental retardation, and psychopathology. *The NADD Bulletin, 2*, 83-87.

Barnhill, J., & Horrigan, J. P. (2002). Tourette's syndrome and autism: A search for common ground. *Mental Health Aspects of Developmental Disabilities, 5*, 7-16.

Beail, N. & Warden, S. (1995). Sexual abuse of adults with learning disabilities. *Journal of Intellectual Disability Research, 39*, 282-287.

Benson, D. F. (1986). Interictal behavior disorders in epilepsy Vol 9. In R. M. Restak (Ed.), *The psychiatric clinics of North America* (pp. 283-292). Philadelphia: W. B. Saunders.

Blumer, D. (1991). Epilepsy and mood disorders. In D. B. Smith, D. M. Treiman, & M. R. Trimble (Eds.), *Advances in Neurology, 55*, 185-196.

Charlot, L.R. (1997). Irritability, aggression and depression in adults with mental retardation: A developmental perspective. *Psychiatric Annals, 27*, 190-197.

Charlot, L.R. (1998). Developmental effects on mental health disorders in person with developmental disabilities. *Mental Health Aspects of Developmental Disabilities, 1*, 30-38.

Dana, L. (1993). Personality disorder in persons with mental retardation. In R. J. Fletcher & A. Dosen (Eds.), *Mental health aspects of mental retardation* (pp. 130-140). New York: Lexington Books.

Day, K. (1994). Male mentally handicapped sex offenders. *British Journal of Psychiatry, 165*, 630-639.

Day, K. (1997). Clinical features and offense behavior of mentally retarded sex offenders: A review of research. *NADD Newsletter, 14*, 86-90.

Deb, S., Matthews, T., Holt, G., & Bouras, N. (2001) *Practice guidelines for the assessment and diagnosis of mental health problems in adults with Intellectual Disability.* Brighton, England: Pavillion.

Dosen, A., & Gielen, J. J. M. (1993). Depression in persons with mental retardation: Assessment and diagnosis. In A. Dosen & R. J. Fletcher (Eds.), *Mental health aspects of mental retardation: Progress in assessment and treatment* (pp. 70-97). New York: Lexington Books.

Edgerton, R. B. (1973). Some sociocultural research considerations. In F. F. De La Cruz & G.D. La Veck (Eds.), *Human sexuality and the mentally retarded* (pp. 240-249). New York: Brunner-Mazel.

Freeman, R. D., Fast, D. K., Burd, L., Kerbeshian, J., Robertson, M. M., & Sandor P. (2000). An international perspective on Tourette syndrome: Selected findings from 3,500 individuals in 22 countries. *Developmental Medicine and Child Neurology, 42*, 436-447.

Gabhard, P. (1973). Sexual behavior of the mentally retarded. In F. F. De La Cruz & G. D. La Veck (Eds.), *Human sexuality and the mentally retarded* (pp. 29-49). New York: Brunner-Mazel.

Gardner, W. I., & Sovner, R. (1994). *Self-injurious behavior.* Willow Street, PA: VIDA Publishing.

Glick, M. (1998). A developmental approach to psychopathology in people with mild mental retardation. In J. A. Burack, R. M. Hodapp, & E.Zigler (Eds.), *Handbook of mental retardation and development* (pp. 563-582). New York: Cambridge University Press.

Harvard Mental Health Letter (2000). Personality disorders – Part I. In L. Grispoon (Ed.), *The Harvard Mental Letter, 16*(9), 1-5.

Jankovic, J. (1997). Phenomenology and classification of tics. *Neurology Clinics, 15*, 267-275.

Lacey, E. P. (1993). Phenomenology of pica. In J. L.Woolston (Ed.), *Child and adolescent clinics of North America: Eating and growth disorders* (pp. 75-91). Philadelphia: W. B. Saunders Co.

Larson, S. A., Lakin, C., Anderson, L., Kwak, N., Lee, J. H., & Anderson, D. (2001). Prevalence of mental retardation and developmental disabilities: Estimate from the 1994/1995 National Health Interview Survey Disability Supplements. *American Journal on Mental Deficiency, 106*, 231-252.

Lowry, M. A. (1998) Assessment and treatment of mood disorders in persons with development disabilities. *Journal of Developmental and Physical Disabilities, 10*, 387-406.

Lumley, V. A., & Miltenberger, R. G. (1997). Sexual abuse prevention for persons with mental retardation. *American Journal on Mental Retardation, 101*, 459-472.

Murphy, W. D., Colman, E. M., & Haynes, M. R. (1983). Treatment and evaluation issues with the mentally retarded sex offender. In J. G. Greer & I. R. Stuart (Eds.), *The sex aggressor: Current perspectives on treatment* (pp. 22-41). New York: Nostrand Rheinhold.

Reiss, S. (1994). Personality disorders. In S. Reiss (Ed.), *Handbook of challenging behavior: Mental health aspects of mental retardation* (pp. 68-73). Worthington, OH: IDS Publishing Corporation.

Rici, D. M. (1993). When mental retardation isn't the only problem. In R. Smith (Ed.), *Children with mental retardation: A parents' guide* (pp. 343-377). Rockville, MD: Woodbine House.

Roberts, J. K. A. (1986). Neuropsychiatric complications of mental retardation Vol 9. In C. Stavrakaki (Ed.), *The psychiatric clinics of North America* (pp. 647-657). Philadelphia: W. B. Saunders.

Rutter, M., Graham, P., & Yule, W. (1970). A *neuropsychiatric study in childhood.* London: Heinemann Medical Books.

Ryan, R. M. (1996). Beam up the universal translator: Interpretation of DSM-IV for persons who use little or no language. In R. M. Ryan (Ed.), *Handbook of mental health care for persons with Developmental Disabilities* (pp. 179-192). Evergreen, CO: S & B Publishing.

Ryan, R. M. (1996). Teach me a new language: Recognizing psychosis in people who do not speak. In R. M. Ryan, *Handbook of mental health care for persons with Developmental Disabilities* (pp. 67-75). Evergreen, CO: S & B Publishing.

Seghorn, T. K., & Ball, C. J. (2000). Assessment of sexual deviance in adults with developmental disabilities. *Mental Health Aspects of Developmental Disabilities, 3*, 47-53.

So, N. K. (1996). Epileptic auras. In E. Wyllie (Ed.), *The treatment of epilepsy: Principles and practice* (pp. 376-384). Baltimore: Williams and Wilkins.

Sovner, R., & Pary, R J. (1993). Affective disorders in developmentally disabled person. In J. L. Matson, & R.P. Barrett, (Eds.), *Psychopathology in the mentally retarded* (2nd ed.). Needham Heights, MA: Allyn & Bacon.

Szymanski, L. S., King, B. H., Goldberg, B., Reid, A., Tonge, B., Cain, N. (1998). Diagnosis of mental disorders. In S. Reiss, & M. G. Aman (Eds.), *Psychotropic medications and Developmental Disabilities: The international consensus handbook* (pp. 3-18). Columbus, OH: Ohio State University Nisonger Center.

Trimble, M. R. (1991). The *psychoses of epilepsy* (pp. 136-150). New York: Raven Press.

Tucker, G. J. (2002). Neuropsychiatric aspects of seizure disorders. In S.C. Yudofsky & R. E. Hales (Eds.), *Textbook of neuropsychiatry and clinical neurosciences* (pp. 673-695). Washington, DC: American Psychiatric Publishing Inc.

Turk, V., & Brown, H. (1994). The sexual abuse of adults with learning disability: Results of a two-year incidence survey. *Mental Handicap Research, 6*, 193-216.

Weisblatt, S. A. (1994) Diagnosis of psychiatric disorders in persons with mental retardation. In N. Bouras (Ed.), *Mental health in mental retardation* (pp. 93-101). Cambridge University Press.

Westen, D., & Shedler, J. (1999). Revising and assessing Axis II, Part II: Toward an empirically-based and clinically-useful classification of personality disorders. *American Journal of Psychiatry, 156*, 273-285.

Wilson, J. G., Lott, R. S., Tsai, L. (1998). Side effects: Recognition and management. In S. Reiss & M.G. Aman (Eds.), *Psychotropic medications and Developmental Disabilities: The international consensus handbook* (pp. 95-114). Columbus, OH: Ohio State University Nisonger Center.

4

Presentation of Mental Disorders in Children and Adolescents with Intellectual Disability

Howard Demb

INTRODUCTION

Young children with Developmental Disabilities (DD) are about three times more likely to have mental disorders as children of average intelligence without DD (Baker, Blacher, Crnic, & Edelbrock, 2002; Tonge, 1999). Estimates of the prevalence of mental disorders in children and adolescents with intellectual disabilities (ID) between ages 3 and 18 years range from 35% to 50%, (Einfeld & Tonge, 1996; Rutter, Tizard, Yule, Graham, & Whitmore, 1976; Stromme & Diseth, 2000) and are as high as 58% in children with both ID and epilepsy (Airaksinen et. al., 2000; Steffenburg, Gillberg, & Steffenburg, 1996). Children with ID demonstrate the same types of mental disorders as children without ID (King, DeAntonia, McCracken, Forness, & Ackerland, 1994). Disorders that occur most often in children with ID include attention-deficit/hyperactivity disorder (ADHD) and other impulse control disorders, opposition defiant disorder (ODD), mood disorders, anxiety disorders, pervasive developmental disorders, stereotypic movement disorders including self-injurious behaviors (SIB) and pica (Pearson et al., 2000; Popper, Gammon, West, & Bailey, 2003; Vanstraelen & Tyrer, 1999). The clinical presentation in children with mild ID is likely to resemble that found in children without ID but, as the level of ID becomes more severe, impaired communication and the consequent difficulties in sharing ideas and emotional experiences often make the clinical picture less clear to the observer (Tonge, 1999). In addition, problems in accurately diagnosing specific mental disorders in children and adolescents with ID reflect the fact that specific symptoms can be one part of more than one diagnostic entity. Thus, problems with attention can be part of ADHD, schizophrenia, bipolar disorder or a pervasive developmental disorder; aggression can be seen in conduct disorders, mood disorders, depression, pervasive developmental disorders or psychosis, and affective instability can be a symptom of a mood disorder but can also be seen in children and adolescents within the autistic spectrum. It is important to look for other behaviors (symptoms) before making a diagnosis of a mental disorder.

Some attempts have been made to describe clusters of behavioral problems of children with ID using standardized symptom questionnaires (Epstein & Cullinan, 1986; Tonge et al., 1996). These clusters have been felt to represent problems involving:

- Aggression and antisocial behavior, for example, fighting, disobedience, disruptiveness;
- Attention disorder, for example, short attention span, distractibility, restlessness, hyperactivity;
- Anxiety, for example, fearfulness, nervousness, crying over minor things, shyness;
- Inferiority, for example, self-consciousness, feelings of inferiority, and
- Social incompetence, for example, social withdrawal, fixed expression, aloofness, self-absorption.

There are several theories about the reasons for the increased risk of psychopathology in children with ID (Volkmar & Dykens, 2002). For example, Weisz (1990) has proposed that the increased risk of experiencing failure in daily living and/or at school may act as a trigger that leads to depression. Nezu & Nezu (1994) suggested that poor communication might lead to increased frustration and disruptive behaviors. Siperstein, Leffort, & Wenz-Gross (1997) point out that behavioral disorders may stem from stressful social interactions including peer rejection, and Greenspan & Granfield (1992) have argued that inappropriate responses to social cues can result in increased isolation. Other investigators have implicated that an increased risk of abuse leads to anxiety and/or depression (Ammerman, Hersen, Van Hasselt, Lubetsky, & Siek, 1994), and that genetic and/or biochemical abnormalities are associated with disorders involving inappropriate behaviors, for example, self-injury (Dykens, 1999).

This chapter will present information about how children and adolescents with ID manifest mental disorders.

DISRUPTIVE BEHAVIOR DISORDERS

Attention-Deficit/Hyperactivity Disorder (ADHD)

Although research has supported the concept of ADHD as a biological condition with a genetic component (Cook et al., 1995; Kado & Takogi, 1996; Pliszka, Carlson, & Swanson, 1999; Barr, 2001; Castellanos et al., 2002), the current diagnostic formulation of this disorder is descriptive and based on reported and observable behaviors. The diagnosis is based on behaviors that are noted before age 7 years, are present in more than one setting, persist for at least six months, and cause either marked distress or significant social or academic impairment (American Psychiatric Association, 2000). It can be diagnosed in individuals with ID as well as those without ID.

Since the diagnostic criteria for ADHD are based on observable behaviors, they can be applied to children and adolescents at all levels of ID and to nonverbal children. There are three different types of ADHD:

- ADHD, Predominantly Inattentive Type: The child is characteristically inattentive, easily distracted, and disorganized but not hyperactive;
- ADHD, Predominantly Hyperactive - Impulsive Type: The child is predominantly fidgety, hyperactive, and impulsive but not inattentive, and

- ADHD, Combined Type (a combination of the first two forms): The child is hyperactive, impulsive and inattentive.

Early signs of ADHD in infancy include sleep disorders, feeding problems (e.g., poor sucking, crying during feedings, or difficulty settling into a comfortable sucking rhythm), irritability, and difficulty calming. Some affected babies may develop self-soothing behaviors such as excessive thumb-sucking, head rolling or banging, or rocking. Once these children begin to crawl they may be in constant motion and oblivious to parental warnings of danger. Such children are often clumsy and accident-prone. Their daily routine is often irregular. As toddlers, they often run instead of walk, and they may seem to be in perpetual motion, often without purpose. By preschool age, they may be prone to intense temper tantrums, may be aggressive, and have difficulty playing cooperatively with others. Difficulties with concentration and remaining seated make it difficult for such children to engage in structured activities. They can be impulsive to a degree that is potentially dangerous as they can hit and/or grab toys from other children without provocation, run into the street, or take objects from stores or other people's homes without a thought about consequences. As they get older, they may enter an ongoing game by barging in without being invited. They frequently lose things, have a hard time organizing their time or activities, and attempt to avoid tasks that take much sustained concentration. They will often run into other children and the resulting pushing or shoving may result in a fight (American Academy of Child and Adolescent Psychiatry, 1998).

While all of the characteristic symptoms of ADHD can be found in children with ID, care must be taken to separate situation-specific inattentiveness, such as at school, if academic expectations are too high, from more generalized inattentiveness. In assessing the meaning of not following through on instructions, one should consider the child's ability to understand language and social rules and whether or not the child has the necessary skills to communicate opposition. When a child takes things, one must consider whether the child has the cognitive ability to understand the consequences of his or her behavior. Similarly, when the child does not respond appropriately to social cues, one must try to determine if the child has the age-appropriate cognitive awareness of what is socially appropriate before trying to interpret the meaning of his or her behaviors.

Example

B. is a 9-year-old boy who was born at six months gestation to a woman that used cocaine during her pregnancy. He weighed one pound. His natural mother was HIV positive, and B. was placed into foster care at age four months. He was described as a jittery and "nervous" infant who was difficult to console. Language development was delayed, and he was only saying a few words when first evaluated at the age of 26 months. At 48 months of age, his cognitive skills were in the mild range of ID, and he was also found to have moderate language impairment. He was adopted at 50 months of age by his original foster mother. Follow-up between the ages of 7 to 10 years resulted in reports of anger and aggressive behaviors at home and in school, and he had difficulty playing cooperatively with others. He would impulsively grab others' toys and fight with other children to keep them. By age 9, he could not concentrate or stay in his seat at school. He began to take methylphenidate (Ritalin) with significant improvement in his behavior.

Oppositional Defiant Disorder (ODD)

This disorder involves a recurrent pattern of behaviors toward authority figures that is:
- Negativistic - stubborn, does not follow directions, not willing to compromise;
- Disobedient and defiant - ignores orders or requests, argues, defies adult rules, blames others for mistakes, and
- Hostile - angry, deliberately annoys others, verbally aggressive, for example, uses foul language (American Psychiatric Association, 2000).

These children are generally viewed as children who "don't listen" and these behaviors are present in multiple settings.

As infants, children who have this disorder are often fussy, colicky, or difficult to soothe. As toddlers and then as pre-schoolers, oppositional temper tantrums can be intense and oppositional episodes often center on sleeping, eating, or toilet-training. These children put things off, or say they have forgotten or not heard the request. Later conflicts center around issues of personal hygiene (e.g., bathing, keeping their room neat) as well as bedtimes and doing homework. These adolescents will also often "answer back". There is little or no ability to take responsibility for their behavior, and they usually blame others for their problems (American Academy of Child and Adolescent Psychiatry, 1998; Loeber, Burke, Lahey, Winters, & Zera, 2000).

Before making such a diagnosis, the clinician must first consider an individual's expressive and receptive language skills and their ability to understand social rules.

Conduct Disorder (CD)

Children and adolescents with a CD have repetitive and persistent patterns of behavior that violate the rights of others and/or age-appropriate social norms or rules (American Psychiatric Association, 2000). These behaviors fall into four main categories:
- Aggression - causing or threatening physical harm to other people or animals;
- Nonaggressive conduct - causing property loss or damage;
- Deceitfulness or theft, and
- Serious violation of rules.

Children with a CD tend to bully or threaten others, often by engaging in fights with the use of weapons, for example, bats and/or knives. Such children may set fires, torture animals, or destroy property. In adolescence they may break into other people's homes or violate rules about curfew, be truant, stay away from home overnight without permission, or even runaway from home (APA, 2000).

Childhood onset CD, which begins before the child is 10 years of age, is often preceded by hyperactivity and is more likely than adolescent onset CD to be persistent. Adolescent onset CD, which is not evident until after the age of ten, is usually accompanied by less aggression and is less likely to persist into adulthood. These adolescents also have more peer friendships than children with childhood onset CD (American Academy of Child and Adolescent Psychiatry, 1998).

Reports of the prevalence of aggression in children without ID vary from 4.3% to 62% depending on the population studied (Booth & Zhang, 1996; Escobar-Chaves et al., 2002; Sosin et al., 1995; Wolke et al., 2000). Aggressive behavior is also a problem in children and adolescents with ID; prevalence rates range from 12% to 45% in different studies

(Bregman, 1991). Aggressive behavior can be associated with a more comprehensive pattern of antisocial behavior as seen in a conduct disorder or can be a violent outburst that is associated with other mental disorders such as depression, bipolar disorder, pervasive developmental disorders, schizophrenia, or anxiety disorders (Sovner & Hurley, 1986).

Here too, when considering the diagnosis of a conduct disorder, the child's ability to understand social rules must be considered. Children with ID who may not experience success in school or in peer interactions may turn to antisocial behaviors as a means to fit in with a peer group or as a means to escape from undesired situations or unwelcome demands (Feinstein & Reiss, 1996).

ANXIETY DISORDERS

Anxiety is the anticipation of future danger or misfortune accompanied by a feeling of unease and/or somatic symptoms such as a stomachache. It is a natural human survival response. The focus can be on an external event or object such as a dog, going to school, or an internal sense of foreboding. Typical symptoms of anxiety include fear, resulting in a sense of discomfort, uneasiness, arousal, and a need to escape.

Anxiety becomes a disorder when the worry or fearfulness is excessive and causes significant distress or impairment in functioning such as in school. Anxiety disorders are characterized by symptoms of sufficient intensity to disrupt social functioning for at least one to six months depending on the disorder (APA, 2000; Barnhill, 1999).

Transitory fears throughout childhood and adolescence are a part of normal development. Newborns fear a loss of support and react to loud noises or novel or unexpected events with over arousal. By 6 months old, there is a fear of strangers that normally persists up to the age of 2 or 3. Fear of separation from parents can begin at age 1 and may persist until 7 or 8 years of age. Preschool children often fear small animals, dark places, changes in the environment, or sleeping alone. Older children may worry about death, examinations, and events in the news such as kidnappings and wars. Teenagers have many worries about social and sexual adequacy (Craske, 1992).

The prevalence of anxiety disorders in the general population is between 3 and 4% (Ford, Goodman, & Meltzer, 2003); while the prevalence of anxiety disorders in children with borderline to moderate ID has been found to be between 10 and 11% (Dekker & Koot, 2003).

Verbal children with ID can sometimes use terms such as "nervousness" or "shakiness" to describe symptoms of anxiety, or they can describe physical sensations of anxiety such as heart pounding or tightness in the chest. Nonverbal children must be observed for physical signs of anxiety such as excessive perspiration, rapid breathing, flushing, chewed fingernails (or toenails), ground down teeth, bitten hands, or a high pulse rate (Ryan, 1996a).

All of the anxiety disorders that affect adults, such as panic disorder, agoraphobia, specific phobias, social phobia, obsessive-compulsive disorder, posttraumatic stress disorder, acute stress disorder, and generalized anxiety disorder (see Chapter 3) can also affect children. Separation anxiety disorder is the only anxiety disorder thought to be specific to childhood and adolescence (APA, 2000).

Separation Anxiety Disorder

According to the DSM-IV-TR (APA, 2000), a diagnosis of separation-anxiety disorder includes developmentally inappropriate and excessive distress, worry, and anxiety whenever there is any separation or suggestion of such from parents or other significant caregivers. A separation-anxiety disorder may be manifested by:
- Difficulty falling asleep when alone;
- Reluctance or refusal to go to sleep without being near a loved one or significant caregiver, or to sleep away from home;
- Recurring nightmares about separation;
- Complaints of physical symptoms (headaches or stomachaches) or vomiting when separation occurs or is anticipated;
- Refusal to be alone without a major attachment figure present;
- Refusal or reluctance to engage in travel training, and
- Refusal or reluctance to go to school.

Although these symptoms are the same for children with and without ID, the key issue has to do with cognitive development. Children with ID may persist in having symptoms of anxiety such as fear of sleeping alone well beyond the chronological age at which this type of behavior would "normally" disappear. It can be a symptom of separation anxiety in an adolescent with mild ID, if it is accompanied by other symptoms less dependent on cognitive development such as a fear of travel training.

Panic Disorder

Panic disorder consists of recurrent panic attacks (a sudden wave of intense apprehension, fearfulness, or terror, with physical symptoms such as shortness of breath, palpations, and chest pains) that occur suddenly, without warning, and often for no apparent reason. In nonverbal children and adolescents the most obvious manifestations of this disorder are the physical symptoms, which may mimic those of a heart attack. Indeed, children or adolescents undergoing a panic attack often think that they are about to die. The prevalence of panic attacks in children with ID is less than 1% (Dekker & Koot, 2003).

Agoraphobia

Agoraphobia is a fear of being in locations or situations (such as crowds, lines, bridges, cars) where escape may be difficult or embarrassing should a panic attack occur, and there is no one there who could help. In children or adolescents with ID, this may manifest itself in a refusal to: leave home, get on a school bus, enter a crowded store, or, get in line in school. The prevalence of agoraphobia in children with ID is 1% (Dekker & Koot, 2003).

Specific (Simple) Phobia

In this disorder exposure to a particular feared object or situation causes substantial anxiety. Subtypes include fears of: specific animals; objects in the natural environment (such as storms, heights, or water); medically related events (such as the sight of blood, injections, injury); specific situations (such as, elevators, enclosed places, bridges); loud sounds, or costumed characters. Observations of a nonverbal child's behaviors in specific situations can often provide sufficient information regarding the presence of a specific phobia. Examples of this would be crying, screaming, kicking and biting when approached with a needle for blood drawing, or falling to the floor and crying when asked to enter an elevator. The prevalence of specific phobias in children with ID is between 6 and 7% (Dekker & Koot, 2003).

Social Phobia

A social phobia involves substantial anxiety caused by certain social situations or performing in front of a group. The most common feared situations are public eating, public speaking, attending parties, using public restrooms, or speaking to authority figures. An otherwise verbal child who does not talk in certain situations, such as school, is said to have selective mutism, a subtype of a social phobia. Children with this type of social phobia often have a mild ID and/or language impairment (Black & Ukde, 1995; Kristensen, 2002). The prevalence of a social phobia in children and adolescents with ID is about 2% (Dekker & Koot, 2003).

Obsessive-Compulsive Disorder (OCD)

To be diagnosed with an obsessive-compulsive disorder (OCD) an individual must have either recurrent, unspoken thoughts (obsessions), uncontrollable repetitive behaviors (compulsions), or both. These must be severe enough to cause a significant impairment in functioning or cause the individual significant anxiety and distress. Examples of obsessions include repeating certain words or numbers in one's head, having recurring thoughts such as "I will hurt someone," or picturing things over and over. Compulsions are actions such as repeated hand-washing or hair-pulling, straightening or organizing things, checking and rechecking, or counting.

Some children recognize that these behaviors and thoughts are senseless or unnecessary. Individuals with ID may not be aware that these symptoms are irrational or strange and do not question the validity of the fears or the compulsive rituals designed to cope with these thoughts. Children with ID who have this disorder may exhibit a number of nonspecific behaviors to indicate their distress. Behaviors such as physical and/or verbal aggression to others, self-injurious behaviors, crying, or being irritable or appearing anxious or nervous should alert the clinician to look for, and ask about, the more specific symptoms of this disorder as noted above (Mesta & Loschen, 1997).

There are those who propose a number of childhood and adult disorders belonging to an obsessive-compulsive (OC) spectrum, which shares features of: compulsivity, impulsivity, harm avoidance, and degrees of insight (Hollander, 1993). Childhood disorders associated with ID, which may fall into this OC spectrum, include impulse control disorders with low degrees of harm avoidance such as trichotillomania (hair-pulling), and autism (Phillips, 2002).

The prevalence of OCD in children and adolescents with ID has been found to be 2.7% (Dekker & Koot 2003).

Posttraumatic Stress Disorder

A posttraumatic stress disorder (PTSD) occurs in some individuals following exposure to an event that involves actual or threatened death or serious injury to themselves or others. It consists of symptoms from each of three clusters involving re-experiencing the event, numbing of general responsiveness with avoidance of stimuli related to the event, and persistent increased arousal. This is associated with feelings of intense fear, helplessness or horror (APA, 2000).

In children, re-experiencing can be seen as manifested in (Scheeringa, Zeanah, Drell, & Larrieu, 1995):
- Re-enactment of the trauma, either directly, such as by attempting to straddle a sibling simulating intercourse, or in play;
- Repeated recollections of the trauma in verbal comments;
- Nightmares, and
- Distress at exposure to reminders of the event;

Numbing is seen in:
- Constriction of play, such as repetitive re-enactment of the trauma with dolls, or repetitive play of a simple nature, such as the arranging of toys in groups without any interaction, or pretend activities among the toys;
- Being socially more withdrawn;
- A restricted range of affect, such as an expressionless or sad face with no modulation by joy, excitement, or loving feelings, and
- A loss of previously acquired skills.

Increased arousal is reflected in:
- Night terrors;
- Night-waking not related to nightmares or night terrors;
- Decreased concentration;
- Hypervigilence, that is, heightened sensitivity and alert to sensory stimuli, and
- Exaggerated startle response.

In children, as with adults, a spectrum of the three clusters exists, so that symptom severity (the number of clusters and the number of symptoms within each cluster exhibited by the child), the nature of the stressor, and the response to the trauma (the child's appraisal of the event and the degree of fear, helplessness or horror experienced by the child) may vary from child to child (Moreau & Zisook, 2002; Sovner, 1986).

In children with or without ID, traumatic events can include: abuse or neglect, with or without consequent foster care placement; witnessing the abuse of a parent; the death of a parent or other loved one; involvement in a serious accident, or the stress involved in trying to cope with impairments in adaptive behaviors (Perry & Polland, 1998). Children with ID are more likely than other traumatized children to have explosive outbursts to perceived threats or as a response to re-experiencing of traumatic events (Pfefferbaum & Allen, 1998). The perception of danger may be related to situations that are reminiscent of earlier abuse or severe stress and may result in new fears.

Symptoms may include:
- Unexplained crying episodes;
- New separation anxiety, fears of the dark, or of toileting;
- Suddenly acting anxious or nervous for no apparent reason;
- Sudden unexplained social withdrawals, or
- Suicidal ideation (Barnhill, 1999; Mester et al., 1997).

Generalized Anxiety Disorder

In generalized anxiety disorder (GAD), there is excessive anxiety and worry, on most days for at least six months. The anxiety and worries may be about a variety of things, including school, upcoming events, or parents' health. There are associated physical symptoms, such as muscle-tension headaches, stomachaches, increased heart rate, or dizziness as well as restlessness, irritability, or sleep disturbances (APA, 2000).

In addition to the symptoms listed above, children with ID and GAD can demonstrate: stereotypies, aggression toward others, self-injurious behaviors, and wariness to a potential environmental threat (Charney et al., 1996; Mester & Loschen, 1997; Schroeda, 1989).

MOOD DISORDERS

Depression

There are two basic forms of depression: major depression (which can occur alone as Major Depressive Disorder or be a part of Bipolar Disorder), a more intense form that must last at least two weeks, and dysthymic disorder, a milder but more chronic form that must last for at least one year in children and adolescents (APA, 2000). Both forms of depression involve a depressed or irritable mood that lasts for most of the day.

Major depressive disorder can involve:
- A loss of interest or pleasure in most activities;
- Feeling tired and lacking energy to engage in most normal activities;
- Eating too little or too much with significant weight loss or weight gain (appetite loss in young children with depression is often accompanied by complaints of stomachaches or headaches);
- Sleeping too little or too much;
- Trouble concentrating or making decisions, or
- Feelings of worthlessness, anger, or guilt that may result in suicidal thoughts or rumination about death.

Depressed mood is said to be more frequent in children with ID than in children without ID. Depressed children are often described as irritable rather than depressed (American Psychiatric Association, 2000). Other characteristics often noted in children with severe to profound ID who are depressed are anger and marked withdrawal. The irritability and anger often results in aggression directed at others or the self (self-injurious behaviors) (Kastner, Friedman, Plummer, Ruiz, & Henning, 1990). The following DSM-IV-TR symptoms of depression can be observed in children and adolescents with ID and limited communication skills (Pawlarcyzk & Beckwith, 1987; Ryan, 1996a; Tsiouris, 2001) (See Chapter 3, Table 3.1.):

- Diminished interests in activities that had been engaged in with pleasure can be observed;
- Weight loss or gain can be documented;
- Recent onset of insomnia or hypersomnia can be observed or reported by caretakers;
- Psychomotor agitation might manifest itself in the form of an increase in activity level or lead to aggression;
- Psychomotor retardation can be reflected by a general slowing of overall functioning or in what caregivers may call sudden "oppositionism" or noncompliance;
- Feelings of worthlessness or guilt may be demonstrated when the child begins to destroy prized possessions or his/her productions such as drawings, with comments that they are "ugly," and
- Diminished ability to concentrate may underlie the difficulties that depressed children with ID have in completing tasks as fast as they had previously.

Example: Depression

K. is a 13-year-old girl who was taken by her father for evaluation as she was argumentative, often uncooperative, and at times seemed sad. Her mother was dying, and a family dog had recently died. She had stopped doing her schoolwork and was said to no longer "listen" to her teachers. She no longer enjoyed playing video games. Her appetite had decreased, and she was beginning to wake up early in the morning. She frequently talked about death.

When interviewed, K. sat quietly with her head down. She looked sad and admitted to feeling sad. She said she felt sad about the death of the family dog and the state of her mother's health. She also reported being angry with teachers whom she said lied about her. She denied suicidal ideation.

Mania

Mania is the other pole of bipolar disorder. DSM-IV-TR (APA, 2000) refers to a distinct period of abnormally elevated, expansive, or irritable mood as a manic episode, if it lasts for at least one week and is accompanied by at least three of the following behaviors:

- Seems grandiose or holds self in high esteem;
- Less need for sleep;
- More talkative than usual;
- Flight of ideas (a nearly continuous flow of accelerated speech with abrupt changes in topic, can be disorganized and incoherent) or subjective experience with racing thoughts;
- Distractibility;
- Increased activity even though it seems appropriate and goal-directed, and

- Over engagement in activities that bring pleasure but have a high risk for painful consequences.

Psychosis may or may not be present. However, there must be the presence of a marked impairment of functioning during a manic episode. For example, a child may decide that he or she is smarter than the teacher and wants to teach the class. As a result, the child is sent to the principal's office as a disciplinary measure. Or, a child who requires little sleep is up at night re-arranging furniture throughout the house and is punished by his parents for awakening them. Or, a child may jump from one task to another at school, and his performance decreases, likely resulting in lower grades.

A hypomanic episode is similar to a manic episode except it is of a shorter duration (at least four days), and there is no marked impairment in functioning.

Bipolar disorders involve manic, hypomanic, and depressive episodes either singly or, in combination and therefore called a mixed episode. DSM-IV-TR lists four subgroups of bipolar disorder:

- Bipolar I: Children who have at least one manic or mixed episode;
- Bipolar II: Children who have at least one episode of major depression and hypomania;
- Cyclothymia: Children who have manifested alternating episodes of hypomania and symptoms of depression that do not meet criteria for a diagnosis of depression, and
- Bipolar disorder not otherwise specified (NOS): Children who do not meet full criteria for any of the other bipolar disorders but suffer from symptoms of a mood disturbance and are functionally impaired.

Children with prepubertal and early adolescent onset bipolar disorder are predominantly irritable, and this disorder is often accompanied by behavior disorders such as ADHD and ODD (Biederman et al., 1996). The clinical course is of a rapid cycling disorder (mania to depression and back again) with little in the way of normal mood states between these episodes of depression and mania (Findling et al., 2001). Adolescent onset bipolar disorder is more likely to have distinct episodes of mania and depression separated by a period of normal mood and more likely to involve symptoms of anxiety (Lewinsoh, Klein, & Seeley, 1995). Longitudinal studies of depressed children and adolescents have shown that at follow-up, 5% to 30% have developed mania or hypomania.

Risk factors for the development of a bipolar disorder are:
- Psychomotor retardation;
- Pharmacologically induced hypomania or mania (usually with an antidepressant), or
- A family history of a bipolar disorder (Birmaher, Arbelaez, & Brent, 2002).

It may be difficult to distinguish between manic symptoms and ADHD in prepubertal children. While there is overlap in the diagnostic criteria for manic episodes of a bipolar disorder and ADHD, five symptoms usually differentiate between the two and are indicative of bipolar disorder:
- Elated mood,
- Grandiosity,

- Racing thoughts/flight of ideas,
- Hypersexuality, and
- Decreased need for sleep (Pavuluri, Naylor, & Janicak, 2002).

Irritability, which is often the predominant mood in childhood mania, is often a common symptom in other forms of childhood psychopathology as well, for example, depression, ADHD, and ODD. However, the type of irritability is different during a manic episode. It is more likely to be intense, involve prolonged temper tantrums (sometimes as long as an hour or more), and lead to violence.

Children and adolescents with ID and bipolar symptoms can show some degree of cognitive disintegration with decreased attention span, impaired memory, or even disorientation, accompanied by a loss of well-established skills, such as dressing and grooming, within a period of a week of the onset of the disorder (McCraken & Diamond, 1998; Sovner, 1986).

Children and adolescents with ID in the manic phase of a bipolar disorder can be assaultative and can be obsessed with knives, using them to threaten people or stabbing them into furniture or the floor. In verbal children with ID, being bossy in an area the child has little knowledge of or no skill in can be evidence of grandiosity. For example, a 7-year-old child with ID, while in a manic episode, began to tell the school bus driver where and when to start, stop, open and close doors etc. Elation can be seen in excitable, silly, giddy behavior with laughing fits and attempts at joking.

Example: Bipolar Disorder

C. was a 14-year-old female with moderate ID and a change in behavior that had begun eight months before her evaluation; prior to that time she had been compliant and sociable. She then became less animated and less social. Her school performance deteriorated, and she spent a considerable amount of time in bed. Her appetite had decreased and she began to lose weight. About four months prior to her evaluation, she began to have one- to two-week periods of irritability, hyperactivity, screaming, decreased sleep, and loss of bowel and bladder control, alternating with two to three weeks of relatively normal functioning. In the week prior to her evaluation, she was described as anxious, irritable, aggressive, and talkative. She would occasionally try to kiss her classmates. There were other episodes of silly behavior such as putting on her younger sister's clothing that did not fit. These behaviors were accompanied by a somewhat elevated mood. C. would also stay up until 2 to 3AM cleaning and straightening up her room.

C.'s history included being born prematurely, having seizures during the neonatal period, and being diagnosed as having mild cerebral palsy. Her development was uniformly delayed. There was a family history of recurrent unipolar depression.

When evaluated, she tended to pace in an agitated fashion. She referred to the examiner as her "boyfriend," and she spoke of other fantasized relationships with a number of different boys. She thought she might be pregnant. She would laugh one moment and become angry and argumentative the next.

PSYCHOSIS AND HALLUCINATIONS

Psychosis is defined as having "delusions or prominent hallucinations" (a perception in the absence of identifiable external stimuli), with the hallucinations occurring in the absence of insight into their pathological nature" (American Psychiatric Association, 2000). A somewhat broader definition would include disorganized speech or grossly disorganized or catatonic behavior (marked motor abnormalities including motoric immobility, excessive seemingly purposeless motor activity, or extreme negativism as in a resistance to be moved). Recently, negative symptoms such as avolition (an inability to initiate and persist in goal-directed activities), decreased motivation, anhedonia (an absence of pleasure from the performance of ordinarily pleasurable acts), and alogia (an impoverishment of thinking inferred from observing speech and language behavior that can be brief or restricted in amount, or can convey little information because it is overly concrete, overly abstract, repetitive or stereotyped) have been included under a broader classification of psychosis (Semper & McClellen, 2003).

Hallucinations are said to be rare in children younger than 6 years of age (Asaad, 1990). They have been reported in 8% of children up to the age of 11 years old in the general population (McGee, Williams, & Poulton, 2000; Schreier, 1999). The presence of hallucinations in children does not automatically signify that the child has a psychosis. In clinical samples of emotionally disturbed but non-psychotic children, hallucinations have been found in individuals as young as 5 years of age (McGee, Williams, & Poulton, 2000; Schreier, 1999). Hallucinations in children between 5 and 13 years of age have been found to be associated with the following mental disorders:
- Acute or chronic anxiety states (including posttraumatic stress disorder),
- Depression,
- Conduct disorder,
- Dissociative disorders,
- Schizophrenic spectrum disorders,
- Mania,
- Intermittent explosive disorders,
- Tourette's disorder, and
- Severe social and psychological deprivation (Burk, DelBeccaro, McCauley, & Clark, 1985; Gerralda, 1984; Schreier, 1999; Ulloa et al., 2000).

They can also be observed as part of neurological conditions such as:
- Migraine, and
- Temporal-lobe epilepsy.

Therefore, hallucinations should be inquired about in a variety of clinical presentations but should be viewed in the context of the rest of the clinical picture, since their presence does not always signify the presence of psychosis.

CHILDHOOD ONSET SCHIZOPHRENIA

Childhood onset schizophrenia is a psychotic disorder that rarely occurs before the age of 7 years. Symptoms of childhood schizophrenia include positive symptoms such as delusions, hallucinations, disorganized speech, grossly disorganized or catatonic behavior, or negative symptoms such as affective flattening, alogia, and abolition. There must be continuous signs of this disturbance present for at least six months, but the signs may be attenuated, such as odd beliefs or unusual (very brief) perceptual experiences instead of delusions or hallucinations, or only the presence of negative symptoms. At least two of the symptoms of schizophrenia must be present for a significant portion of one month. If the delusions are bizarre, such as a visitor from another planet eating one's organs from inside of one's body, or the hallucinations involve voices "commenting or conversing," then the presence of only one item is required. The continuous signs of disturbance must include marked deterioration of functioning or, in the case of young children, failure to achieve expected levels of social development such as the ability to tolerate separation and attend school. The majority of children with childhood schizophrenia present with auditory hallucinations, delusions, and disorganized speech or behavior (See below.) (Russell, Bott, & Sammons, 1989; Sporn & Rapport, 2001).

Children with mild to moderate ID can usually be diagnosed as having schizophrenia using standard DSM-IV-TR criteria for schizophrenia (American Psychiatric Association, 2000; Lee, Friedlander, & Donnelly, 1998). A detailed developmental history can provide evidence of a change (deterioration) in behavior and level of functioning. Evidence of hallucinations can be obtained from a verbal child. Auditory hallucinations of a "commenting" type are most common. Hallucinations in children with ID can be of the command type (voices telling them to do something such as hurt themselves or someone else) or of the conversing or commenting type (a voice telling the child that he/she is "stupid" or "ugly"). Visual hallucinations can be reported or, in the case of a nonverbal child, can be inferred by behaviors such as the child looking at the corner of the room as if something were there, or attempting to strike out at or punch the air, as if there were someone there to hit. Delusional thinking is most often persecutory, for example, thinking people are going to do harm or thinking food is being poisoned. In nonverbal children such delusions may be inferred when a child, who is not depressed, stops eating, or a child who is not otherwise frightened begins to scream whenever he/she must pass a clothing closet. Verbal children can manifest a formal thought disorder by manifesting loose associations (unrelated ideas that are randomly expressed) or by engaging in conversations, which lack cohesion, such as failing to tie together ideas in a coherent fashion.

What follows are examples of thought disorders in children with ID:
- A. is a 5-year-old boy with ID who was asked how a knife and a scissors were the same? He replied "The same. They are not talking. They look like a grape, like a purple grape." When asked, "What can we put water in and drink out of?" he replied, "The water is just like a cat." He also spontaneously stated, "I pooped. I'm going to poop on the Ferris wheel because there is a belly in there."
- B. is a 7-year-old boy with ID. While looking at a picture of a knife and bread he said, "The bread got cut on the knife with the eye. The eye went over and the eye went crossed. The knife cut the eye, and the eye cut him back. He cut everything

that he cuts. He cut the bread and two toes, and he cooked it and no one. They were a family."

- C. is a 6-year-old girl with borderline ID. When asked if her ears ever played tricks on her she said, "Yes. I hear anybody and I go outside to play football and basketball. I go to the park. My dad takes me. He takes my sister and brother and me. I like dogs. I hate cats. Cats scratch me. Dogs be nice. I watch TV. My favorite color is pink, blue, green, and black."

It is not easy to assess a thought disorder in a child with limited or no language. However, negative symptoms such as affective flattening, a decrease in attention and concentration, or inappropriate affect can also be observed (Lee et al., 1998; Ryan, 1996b).

Example: Childhood Schizophrenia

A. was a 9-year-old boy with mild ID who had a history of jaundice following birth. He was treated with phototherapy. He was a colicky infant who slept irregularly. Pediatric evaluations during his first two years of life revealed signs of generalized hypotonia (a muscle tone). He sat at 9 months, never crawled, and did not walk until 27 months old. He began to use single words at about 24 months. Hyperactivity was noted by the age of 3, and he became destructive at about the age of four. When he was 5 years old, he began to hit walls while vocalizing. These behaviors were noted in kindergarten, and by the second grade he began to appear anxious and withdrawn but would occasionally attack children whom he accused of cursing and teasing him. By the third grade, his motivation and functioning in school began to decline, and he began to have problems falling and staying asleep. He appeared to be anxious and depressed and withdrew socially as he began to spend most of his time in his room where he was noted to stare into space while talking to himself. He was referred for an evaluation when he walked over to a classroom window and said that he could fly. When seen for the evaluation, he reported that there was a little man inside of his head that talked to him and told him to do "bad things."

PERVASIVE DEVELOPMENTAL DISORDERS (AUTISTIC SPECTRUM DISORDERS)

Pervasive developmental disorder (PDD) or autistic spectrum disorders (Ozonoff, Rogers, & Hendren, 2003) are among the most severe developmental disorders and involve disorders of social, language, emotional, and often cognitive domains. These disorders are listed in DSM-IV-TR (American Psychiatric Association, 2000) as mental disorders with emphasis on the disorder as one of impaired development.

The PDD category is also referred to as an autistic spectrum because the manifestations of social, communication, and other problems vary widely in type and severity. As a result, many different combinations of impairments are observed. The currently recognized PDD disorders include: autistic disorder (autism); Asperger's disorder; Rett's disorder, childhood disintegrative disorder; and PDD Not Otherwise Specified (PDD NOS). ID is present in between 40% and 55% of young children with PDD NOS and is present in about 77% of children with an autistic disorder (Mesibov, Adams, & Klinger, 1997; Sigman, Dissanayake, Arbelle, & Ruskin, 1997)). An exception is Asperger's disorder, where speech is less commonly delayed, and most individuals with this disorder function within the average range of intelligence (Wing, 1981; Wing, 1991). In one sample of 12 children with Asperger's disorder, the average full scale IQ was 115 (Ozonoff, South, & Miller, 2000) while in another sample of 35 children there was no child with a full scale IQ less than 70 (Manjiviona & Prior, 1999). Children with ID and PDD have significant impairments in reciprocal social interaction and social communication (either verbal or nonverbal). A common mistake has been to diagnose a PDD in people with ID who present with a speech delay and self-stimulatory behavior. Such individuals are usually able to engage in interpersonal, reciprocal interaction and in interpersonal communication, appropriate to their developmental level. Therefore, when one is considering the diagnosis in an individual who exhibits self-stimulatory behaviors, the diagnosis of a PDD should not be made unless this individual also has significant impairments in social skills and social communication for their developmental level.

Severe mental/developmental conditions tend to co-occur with other developmental, mental, or medical conditions. In the case of PDD these conditions can involve symptoms such as hyperactivity, obsessive-compulsive phenomena, perceptual abnormalities, self-injury, stereotypy, tics, affective symptoms, or anxiety (Volkmar, Klin, & Cohen, 1997). Many of these symptoms can, and sometimes do, warrant a comorbid diagnosis. For example, tics can be diagnosed as a tic disorder or Tourette's disorder; obsessive compulsive behaviors can be diagnosed as an obsessive-compulsive disorder; children with associated perceptual abnormalities can be diagnosed as having childhood schizophrenia (Sverd, Dubey, Schweitzer & Ninan, 2003), or a specific anxiety disorder or mood disorder can be diagnosed. Despite the fact that ADHD remains an exclusionary criteria for a diagnosis of autism (AD) (APA 2000), there are those who feel that when a child has ADHD-like symptoms that meet criteria for that diagnosis, the diagnosis should be made in a child with any of the PDDs (Frazier et al., 2001; Goldstein & Schweback, 2002). Since many of these symptoms have been described as "associated features" of autism or other PDDs (American Psychiatric Association, 2000) the decision to add a comorbid diagnosis is not easy and may depend upon whether or not the symptoms meet DSM-IV criteria for the disorder, the severity of the associated condition, or the availability of an appropriate treatment modality for the comorbid condition.

Autism is discussed in detail in Chapter 6. Only a brief overview will be provided here.

Autistic Disorder (Autism)

A diagnosis of autistic disorder (AD) requires that at least 6 of 12 criteria be met, including at least two of the first subgroup (qualitative impairment in social interaction), at least one of the second subgroup (qualitative impairment in interpersonal communication), and at least one of the third subgroup (restricted, repetitive, and stereotyped patterns of behavior, interests, and activities) (American Psychiatric Association, 2000). The child must display these delays and abnormal functioning before 3 years of age. Before making the diagnosis one must be certain that the symptoms are inherent in the individual rather than reactions to the immediate situation.

Since impairments in social interactions are central to the diagnosis of autism, it must be clear that these impairments are not the same as shyness or avoiding others. Shy or avoidant children avoid social situations where they fear that they may be embarrassed, and when exposed to these situations, they feel anxious. Even when the fear is excessive or unreasonable, shy or avoidant children may not recognize this. Children with AD, on the other hand, fail to establish friendships either because, when young, they have little or no interest in other children as being socially rewarding, or because, when older, and when there is some interest, they lack an understanding of the conventions of the types of ordinary social interactions necessary to initiate or maintain a friendship. This lack of understanding may result in an elevated level of anxiety about entering into a social situation, but the anxiety is probably driven by confusion or uncertainty about how to interact rather than a fear of embarrassment.

Asperger's Disorder

It is not clear whether Asperger's disorder is a condition distinct from autism (Klin & Volkmar, 2002; Volkmar & Klin, 2000). Asperger's disorder usually involves no cognitive or psychomotor developmental delay. The deficit in social and emotional interaction, although present, seems to be less severe than in individuals with AD (Wing, 1981). Individuals who are felt to have Asperger's disorder tend to have communication difficulties marked by being monotonic and pedantic (talking too long in too much detail about topics of limited interest to others such as maps, trains, the weather). They also lack empathy and engage in one-sided social interactions during which they may make inappropriate comments that may alienate the listener. They may also be more moralistic and rule bound than individuals with AD (Rosenn, 1999). Clumsiness and poor handwriting is more frequent in Asperger's disorder than in AD. When stressed, children or adolescents with Asperger's disorder can become oppositional or aggressive and engage in tantrums or rages referred to as "meltdowns." (Smith, 2003) Prognosis concerning independence and professional skills is usually better than in AD, but people with Asperger's disorder occasionally demonstrate psychotic episodes earlier in life. It is suggested that the differences between Asperger's disorder and AD represent variations in a spectrum of clinical features of the same neurobiological deficit, with a milder impairment in the former.

Childhood Disintegrative Disorder

Childhood disintegrative disorder (CDD) is a condition marked by a striking deterioration in multiple areas of development after a prolonged period of normal development (American Psychiatric Association, 2000). The condition is accompanied by the development of various features seen in AD, such as social disturbances, stereotypic movements, loss of interest in the environment, and resistance to change (Malhotra & Gupta, 1999). The onset is usually between the second and fourth year of life, and the neurologic regression can be gradual or abrupt. The regression can last from four to eight weeks (Ozonoff & Rogers, 2003) or can progresses for many years, usually resulting in a state of severe ID (Volkmar, Klin, Marans, & Cohen, 1997). Some individuals have preservation of motor skills in spite of cognitive deterioration.

CDD differs from AD in that in AD developmental abnormalities are usually noted in the first two years of life, whereas in CDD the symptoms are preceded by at least two years of normal development. Also, unlike AD, there is little developmental growth over time. Therefore, CDD should be considered when a child, whose development was entirely normal for months or years, loses the previously acquired skills and exhibits behavioral changes (Volkmar & Rutter, 1995).

TABLE 4.1
Types of Attachment Disorders

Type	Description
Non-attached	Lack of preference for a particular adult caregiver Emotionally withdrawn and unattached
Indiscriminate/Disinhibited/Diffuse Attachments	Wanders off, socially promiscuous, friendly Overtures and seeks nurturance from unfamiliar adults Risk-taking and accident prone
Inhibited Attachment	Readily withdraws from social interactions with people other than attachment figure (AF) Reluctance to play with toys when with unfamiliar people Restricted range of affect Can be excessively clinging or compliant with AF Can be frightened of AF or frightened in the absence of the AF
Aggressive/Coercive Attachment	Angry outbursts toward AF or the self Can threaten or reject Can behave seductively disarming, coy, or helpless
Anxious/Depressed	Panics during separation Displays sad affect Unfocused behavior
Role-reversal Attachment	Assumes parental roles Can be bossy and controlling during interaction with AF

Rett's Disorder

Rett's disorder is a disorder that affects mainly females (Tsi, 1994). Individuals with Rett's disorder have apparently normal development until the age of 5 to 18 months. Then the neurologic acquisitions stop and later regress. There are losses of meaningful hand movements between the age of 5 and 30 months with the appearance of stereotyped midline gestures resembling handwringing, twisting, or washing. Females with Rett's disorder rarely have self-injurious behavior, and the repertoire of stereotypic movements is usually restricted to handwringing without variation in form or speed. Between 5 and 48 months of age there is a simultaneous deceleration of head growth resulting in a small head size, known as acquired microcephaly. Other signs include epilepsy, teeth-grinding, and deeper and more rapid breathing than normal. Important motor and cognitive impairment develops between 2 and 4 years of age. There is social isolation, the absence of language (or other nonverbal communication), and behavioral changes. Later on, the child begins to have difficulty coordinating muscles needed for voluntary purposeful movements of the trunk, and progressive scoliosis develops. Progressive weakness occurs in all four limbs, and motor skills tend to be lost (Szymanski et al., 1998). Recovery of communication is quite limited, but there may be some small developmental gains and some increased interest in the social environment may be noted in late childhood or early adolescence (APA 2000).

Pervasive Developmental Disorder Not Otherwise Specified (PDD NOS)

The diagnosis of PDD NOS is considered when the individual does not meet all of the required diagnostic criteria for any of the PDDs, or the onset is after the age of 3. A category similar to PDD NOS is included in ICD-10 under the label of atypical autism (World Health Organization, 1992). Neither PDD NOS nor atypical autism has a clear definition.

ATTACHMENT DISORDERS

Attachment is a biologically based motivational system that evolves during the first several years of life and motivates the young child to seek comfort, support, and nurturance from specific attachment figures. According to attachment theory, the child uses the attachment figure as a secure base from which to venture out and explore as well as a safe haven to return to in time of danger (Bowlby, 1982).

A mental age is the chronological age at which a performance or behavior is "average" or "normal". With regard to attachment, we will use this term to mean the chronological age when most children achieve a developmental level.

Preferred or focused attachment is not evident at birth. From a mental age of approximately 2 to 3 month's old, infants respond to a wide variety of people, not showing a strong preference for a single attachment figure. From mental ages of 2 to 3 months to about 7 months, infants tend to discriminate more with regard to social responsiveness and by a mental age of 9 or 10 months, show a clear preference for certain persons. Stranger wariness and separation protest begin to appear between mental ages of 8 to 12 months, and until about the mental age of 3 years, the child will tend to resist separation from the attachment figure, return to the attachment figure for support and comfort, and use the attachment figure as a base from which to engage in non-attachment behaviors such as play and exploration (Brazelton, Kowslowski, & Main, 1974; Simpson, 1999).

The "strange situation" procedure is a laboratory procedure used to classify attachments (Ainsworth, Blehar, Waters, & Wall, 1978). The procedure involves a series of interactions including separation and reunion between a young child, an attachment figure, and a stranger. There are eight episodes and the first begins with the mother and child entering and exploring the interview room. Next, there is the introduction of a stranger who begins to play with the child; the parent then leaves the child with the stranger (first separation) and later returns as the stranger leaves (first reunion). The parent then leaves the child alone in the room (second separation) and the stranger returns without the parent. The final episode involves the mother returning (second reunion) and the stranger leaving. Based upon the child's reactions to the separations (such as little visible distress, signs of missing the parent, quite distressed) and the reunions (such as greetings, smiling, looking away, seeking distance from the parent, anger, rejection), the child can be classified as having a specific type of attachment.

The child's attachment relationship to a particular caregiver is classified as secure or as one of several types of insecure attachments, at different developmental levels. In children with mental ages between 18 and 36 months the insecure attachments are described as being either avoidant, resistant, or disorganized, while in children with mental ages between 36 and 60 months, the insecure attachments are described as being either avoidant, dependent, controlling, or insecure. Other proposed types of attachment disorders include: nonattached (a failure to develop a preferred attachment figure), indiscriminate or diffuse, inhibited (unwilling to venture away from their attachment figure), aggressive (a relationship marked by anger and frustration), and role-reversed or controlling (where the child is either overly nurturing or overly bossy).

DSM-IV-TR characterizes disorders of attachment as being a result of (reactive to) "pathogenic care," such as disregard for the child's physical or emotional needs (maltreatment) or frequent changes of primary caregivers. This reactive attachment disorder of infancy or early childhood must begin before the age of 5 years, cannot solely be the result of a developmental delay or a PDD, and must be associated with "pathogenic care". It is characterized by markedly disturbed and developmentally inappropriate social relatedness in most contexts such as the child's excessive inhibition, a demonstrated resistance to being comforting, or manifesting indiscriminate sociability by excessive familiarity with relative strangers (APA, 2000). Though there are several classifications of attachment disorder, not all presume "pathogenic care" as an antecedent event (Boris, Zeanah, Larrieu, Scheeringa, & Heller, 1998). These are not DSM-IV-TR classifications and are listed in Table 4.1.

It is felt that affected children should have a mental age of at least 10 months so that failure to demonstrate a preferred attachment would not be due to cognitive limitations (Zeanah & Boris, 2000). While, in general, there have been few, and only modest, associations between attachment classifications and global measures of intelligence, the disinhibited/indiscriminate attachment disorder is common in children with ID, and a diagnosable mental disorder without any evidence of "pathogenic care" (Thompson, 1999).

Tics/Tourette's Disorder

Tics are rapid, sudden, intermittent, non-rhythmic, recurrent, involuntary, or semi-voluntary movement (motor tics) or sounds (vocal tics). Tics are the hallmark of Tourette's disorder, a movement disorder characterized by the presence of multiple motor and vocal tics with the average age of onset at about 6 or 7 years (Freeman et al., 2000).

Tourette's disorder is accompanied by ID in about 4% of the cases (range 1% to 14% in various studies) (Freeman et al., 2000). It is a chronic disorder with a variable and fluctuating course, which usually worsens in pre-adolescence, but by the age of 18 one half of the persons with Tourette's disorder are free of tics (Jankovic, 2001). Tourette's disorder usually starts with facial tics (eye-blinking or grimaces) and progresses to motor tics, sometimes as complex stereotyped or purposeful movements. Vocal tics include grunts, words, or phrases. Echolalia (repeating what someone has said) or coprolalia (foul language) can be present. Motor and vocal tics are often preceded by premonitory sensations such as localized feelings of discomfort. These sensations are temporarily relieved by the execution of the tic (Leckman, Walker, Goodman, Pauls, & Cohen, 1994). In clinical samples, children with the disorder also frequently have behavioral symptoms that are symptomatic of an attention-deficit/hyperactivity disorder or an obsessive-compulsive disorder (Walkup, Scahill, & Riddle, 1995; Zohar et al., 1997). Self-injurious behaviors (SIB), sleep disorders, and anger-control problems are also more common in those individuals with Tourette's disorder that are seen in mental health clinics (Allen, Singer, Brown, & Salam, 1992; Budman, Bruun, Park, & Olson, 1998; Robertson, 1992), but there is a very low rate of behavioral problems in individuals with Tourette's disorder in the general population who do not seek mental health services (Freeman et al., 2000).

Feeding and Eating Disorders

Some of the eating disorders listed in DSM-IV-TR (APA, 2000) include:
- Anorexia Nervosa, defined as a refusal to maintain a minimally normal body weight, a fear of gaining weight, and a significant disturbance in the perception of shape or size of one's body;
- Bulimia Nervosa, defined as binge eating or inappropriate compensatory methods (such as inducing vomiting) to prevent weight gain (both symptoms must occur an average of at least twice each week for three months), and
- Eating Disorder Not Otherwise Specified.

These disorders may not be more common in children and adolescents with ID than in children and adolescents with average cognitive abilities, but feeding problems are frequently reported as problem areas in children with physical motor impairment and cognitive behavioral impairment (Wolke, Meyer, Ohrt, & Riegel, 1995). There are no universally accepted guidelines to determine when a feeding problem becomes a disorder (Benoit, 2000). However, food refusal associated with texture sensitivity, problem with muscle control of the mouth and tongue, and/or resistance to change are often seen in children with ID. Rigid habits based on food texture tend to fall into two main categories: dry foods (crispy, crunchy) and soft foods (mushy). In some cases, an infringement on the sometimes restricted repertoire of foods serving to make up the child's core diet can be met with food refusal, or, in extreme cases, temper tantrums, retching, or vomiting.

Infants and young children may ingest inedible substances (pica) such as paint, plaster, string, hair, or cloth in a voluntary or stereotyped fashion. Older children eat animal droppings, sand, insects, leaves, or pebbles (APA, 2000). Adolescents and adults consume clay or soil (Lacey, 1993). (See Chapter 3 for more information). Moderate to severe ID is a predisposing factor for rumination, the regurgitation and re-chewing of food. This occurs with greater frequency as the severity of the ID increases (American Academy of Child and Adolescent Psychiatry, 1999).

Sleep Problems and Disorders

Newborns have sleep and periods awake that occur randomly across a 24-hour day. By 3 months there should be a clear differentiation between day and night, so that they sleep more at night and are awake more during the day. By 6 months most infants sleep through the night (Anders, Goodlin-Jones, & Sadeh, 2000).

Studies of sleep problems in children with ID reveal that the most common sleep problems are settling (sleep onset) and waking (sleep maintenance), while there are also frequent reports of early awakening (Quine, 1991). Challenging behaviors (such as aggression, self-injury, screaming, temper tantrums, and non-compliance) are present more often in children with ID and sleep problems than in children with ID but without sleep problems. Sleep disturbance in young people with ID are often associated not only with behavior disturbances but also with attendant maternal stress and difficulties with family functioning (Wigg & Stores, 1996).

The prevalence of sleep problems in children with ID and behavior problems has been reported to be as high as 88% and as low as 34% (Clements, Wing, & Dunn, 1986; Jan, Freeman, & Fast, 1999; Piazza, Fisher, & Kahng, 1996). Reported sleep problems tend to decrease with age, as 56% of children with disabilities under the age of 6, 31% of 5 to 10 year olds, and 28% of 10 to 15 year olds were reported to have sleep problems (Clements et al., 1986).

DSM-IV-TR describes sleep disorders as "primary," if they are not a result of a mental disorder, a general medical condition, or substance use. Primary sleep disorders are presumed to arise from abnormalities in sleep-wake generating or timing mechanisms. Primary sleep disorders are subdivided into dyssomnias and parasomnias. The dyssomnias are characterized by abnormalities in the amount, quality, or timing of sleep.

The dyssomnias include:
- Primary insomnia (trouble falling asleep);
- Primary hypersomnia (excessive sleepiness);
- Narcolepsy (irresistible attacks of refreshing sleep during the day associated with either brief episodes of sudden bilateral loss of muscle tone, or hallucinations or paralysis at the beginning or end of sleep episodes);
- Breathing-related sleep disorder (a sleep disruption caused by a sleep-related breathing condition such as an airway obstruction), or
- Circadian-rhythm sleep disorder (most often caused by work schedules that result in a mismatch between when a person is allowed to fall asleep and his/her biological sleep-wake schedule).

The parasomnias are characterized by abnormal behavioral or biological events occurring in association with sleep or sleep-wake transitions.

The parasomnias include:
- Nightmares;
- Sleep terrors (abrupt awakening from sleep associated with intense fear, and often not responsive to parental effort to comfort), and
- Sleepwalking.

Sleep-walking, sleep-talking, and night terrors (which are associated with partial arousal from sleep) as well as head-banging (which occurs with sleep onset), and nightmares (which occur during REM sleep) are all present in children and adolescents with ID. Teeth-grinding (bruxism) is also reported as a sleep-related phenomenon in children with ID (Poindexter, 1998).

Treatment

The basic principles of treatment for a given mental disorder are essentially the same for children and adolescents with or without ID (American Academy of Child and Adolescent Psychiatry, 1999). However, treatment approaches require modification in keeping with the individual's cognitive limitations, communication skills, and life circumstances (Harris, 2001). Details about treatment can be found in Chapters 7 and 9.

SUMMARY

There seems to be general agreement that the same principles that apply to the diagnosis of children and adolescents in the general population, apply to children and adolescents with cognitive limitations. The diagnostic process, as usual, involves obtaining information from parents and/or other caregivers as well as direct observations of the child or adolescent in one or more settings. When dealing with a nonverbal child or adolescent, inferences must often be made about the meaning of a behavior, such as postulating auditory or visual hallucinations in a nonverbal child who looks off to a corner of the room and begins to look frightened or laugh inappropriately. Enough symptoms (behaviors) can usually be observed directly to meet the criteria for a particular mental disorder (Castellanos et al., 1996; King, State, Shah, Davanzo, & Dykens, 1997).

In view of the difficulties in making an accurate diagnosis in some children and adolescents with ID, clinicians in this field are looking forward to new approaches to the diagnosis of mental disorders. These include neuroimaging (Botteron, 2001; King et al., 1997; Reba 1993; Salimpoor, 2003), and research in genetics (Rena & El-Mallakah, 1997; Sutcliffe & Nurmi, 2003; Veenstra-Vanderweele & Cook, 2003), including attempts to discover whether certain behavioral or cognitive characteristics can be attributed to a particular gene or chromosome (a "behavioral phenotype") (Hodapp & Dykens, 2001; Hudzik, 2001).

REFERENCES

Ainsworth, M. D. S., Blehar, M. S., Waters, E., & Wall, S. (1978). Patterns of Attachment: *A psychological study of the strange situation.* Hillsdale, NJ: Lawrence Erlbaum.

Airaksinen, E. M., Matilainen, R., Mononen, T., Mustonen, K., Partanen, J., Jokela, V., et al. (2000). A population-based study on epilepsy in mentally retarded children. *Epilepsia, 41,* 1214-1220.

Allen, R. P. Singer, H. S., Brown, J. E., & Salam, M. M. (1992). Sleep disorders in Tourette syndrome: A primary or unrelated problem? *Pediatric Neurology, 8,* 275-280.

American Academy of Child and Adolescent Psychiatry (1998). Disruptive Behavior Disorders. In D. B. Pruitt (Ed.), *Your Child: What Every Parent Needs to Know about Childhood Development from Birth to Preadolescence* (pp. 335-353). New York: Harper Collins Publishers, Inc.

American Academy of Child and Adolescent Psychiatry (1999). Practice parameters for the assessment and treatment of children, adolescents, and adults with autism and other pervasive developmental disorders. *Journal of the American Academy of Child and Adolescent Psychiatry, 38*(Suppl.), 32S-54S.

American Psychiatric Association (2000). *Diagnostic and Statistical Manual of Mental Disorders,* (Rev. 4th ed.). Washington, DC: American Psychiatric Association.

Ammerman, R. T., Hersen, M., Van Hasselt, V. B., Lubetsky, M. J., & Siek, W. R. (1994). Maltreatment in psychiatrically hospitalized children and adolescents with Developmental Disabilities: Prevalence and correlates. *Journal of the American Academy of Child and Adolescent Psychiatry, 33*, 567-576.

Anders, T., Goodlin-Jones, B., & Sadeh, A. (2000). Sleep disorders. In C. H. Zeanah, Jr. (Ed.), *Journal of Infant Mental Health* (2nd ed., pp. 326-339). New York: The Guilford Press.

Asaad, G. (1990). *Hallucinations in clinical psychiatry: A guide for mental health professionals* (pp. 86-94). New York: Brunner/Mazel Inc.

Baker, B. L., Blacher, J., Crnic, K. A., & Edelbrock, C. (2002). Behavior problems and parenting stress in families of 3-year-old children with and without developmental delays. *American Journal on Mental Retardation, 107*, 433-444.

Barnhill, L. J. (1999). Diagnosis and treatment of anxiety disorders in persons with developmental disabilities. *The NADD Bulletin, 2*, 110-115.

Barr, C. L. (2001). Genetics of Childhood disorders: XXII, ADHD, Part 6: The dopamine D_4 receptor gene. *Journal of the American Academy of Childhood Adolescent Psychiatry, 40*: 118-121.

Benoit, D. (2000). Feeding disorders, failure to thrive and obesity. In C. H. Zeanah, Jr. (Ed.), *Handbook of infant mental health* (2nd ed., pp. 339-352). New York: The Guilford Press.

Biederman, J., Faraone, S., Mick, E., Wozniak, J., Chen, L., Ouellette, C., et al. (1996). Attention-deficit hyperactivity disorder and juvenile mania: An overlooked comorbidity? *Journal of the American Academy of Child and Adolescent Psychiatry, 35*, 997-1008.

Birmaher, B., Arbelaez, C., & Brent, D. (2002). Course and outcome of child and adolescent major depressive disorder. In G. A. Carlson & J. H. Kashani (Eds.), *Child and Adolescent Clinic of North America:* Vol. 11. *Mood Disorders* (pp. 619-637). Philadelphia: W. B. Saunders Co.

Black, B. & Uhde, T. W. (1995). Psychiatric characteristics of children with selective mutism: A pilot study. *Journal of the American Academy of Child and Adolescent Psychiatry, 34*, 847-855.

Boris, N. W., Zeanah, C. H., Larrieu, J.A., Scheeringa, M. S., & Heller, S. S. (1998). Attachment disorders in infancy and early childhood: A preliminary investigation of diagnostic criteria. *American Journal of Psychiatry, 155*, 295-297.

Botteron, K. N. (2001). Genetic analysis of brain-imaging abnormalities. In R. D. Todd (Ed.), *Child and Adolescent Psychiatric Clinics of North America:* Vol. 10. *Genetic Contributions to Early Onset Psychopathology* (pp. 241-258). Philadelphia: W. B. Saunders Co.

Bowlby, J. (1982). *Attachment and Loss,* (Vol. 1: 2nd ed.) New York: Basic Books.

Brazelton, T. B., Kowslowski, B., & Main, M. (1974). The origins of reciprocity: The early mother-infant interaction. In M. Lewis, L. A. Rosenbaum (Eds.), *The Effects of Infants on Its Caregiver* (pp. 196-222). New York: John Wiley & Sons.

Bregman, J. (1991). Current developments in the understanding of mental retardation: Part II. *Journal of the American Academy of Child and Adolescent Psychiatry, 30*, 861-872.

Budman, C. L., Bruun, R. D., Park, K. S., & Olson, M. E. (1998). Rage attacks in children and adolescents with Tourette's disorder: A pilot study. *Journal of Clinical Psychiatry, 59,* 576-580.

Burk, P., DelBeccaro, M., McCauley, E., & Clark, C. (1985). Hallucinations in children. *Journal of the American Academy of Child Psychiatry, 24,* 71-75.

Castellanos, F. X., Giedd, J. N., Marsh, W. L., Hamburger, S. D., Vaituzio, A. C., Dickstein, et al. (1996). Quantitative brain magnetic resonance imaging in attention-deficit hyperactivity disorder. *Archives of General Psychiatry, 53,* 607-616.

Castellanos, F. X., Lee, P. P., Sharp, W., Jeffries, N. O., Greenstein, D. K., Clasen, L. S., et al. (2002). Developmental trajectories of brain volume abnormalities in children and adolescents with attention-deficit/hyperactivity disorder. *Journal of the American Medical Association, 288,* 1740-1748.

Charney, D. S., Nagy, L., Bremer, D., Goodard, A. W., Yehuda, R., & Southwich, S. (1996). Neurobiology mechanisms of human anxiety. In B. S. Fogel, R. B. Schiffer, & S. M. Rao (Eds.), *Neuropsychiatry* (pp. 257-272). Baltimore: Williams and Wilkins.

Clements, J. Wing, J., & Dunn, G. (1986). Sleep problems in handicapped children: A preliminary study. *Journal of Child Psychology and Psychiatry, 27,* 399-407.

Cook, E. H., Jr., Stein, M. A., Krasowski, M. D., Cox, N. J., Olkon, D. M., Kieffer, J. E., et al. (1995). Association of attention-deficit disorder and the dopamine transporter gene. *American Journal of Human Genetics, 56,* 993-998.

Craske, M. G. (1992). Fear and anxiety in children and adolescents. *Bulletin of the Menninger Clinic, 61*(Suppl. A), (2) A4-A36.

Dekker, M., & Koot, H. M. (2003). DSM IV disorders in children with borderline to moderate intellectual disability, I: Prevalence and impact. *Journal of the American Academy of Child and Adolescent Psychiatry, 42,* 915-922.

Dykens, E. M. (1999). Direct effect of genetic mental retardation syndromes: Maladaptive behavior and psychopathology. *International Review of Research in Mental Retardation, 22,* 1-26.

Einfeld, S. I., & Tonge, B. J. (1996). Population prevalence of psychopathology in children and adolescents with intellectual disability. II Epidemiological findings. *Journal of Intellectual Disability Research, 40*(2), 99-109.

Epstein, M. H., & Cullinan, D. (1986). Patterns of maladjustment among mentally retarded children and youth. *American Journal of Mental Deficiency, 91,* 127-134.

Feinstein, C. & Reiss, A. L. (1996). Psychiatric disorders in mentally retarded children and adolescents: The challenges of meaningful diagnosis. In F.R. Volkmar (Ed.), *Child and Adolescent Clinics of North America: Vol. 5. Mental Retardation* (pp. 827-852). Philadelphia: W. B. Saunders Co.

Findling, R. L. Gracious, B. L. McNamara, N. K., Youngstrom, E. A., Demeter, C.A., Branicky, L. A., et al. (2001). Rapid, continuous cycling and psychiatric comorbidity in pediatric bipolar I disorder. *Bipolar Disorder, 3,* 202-210.

Ford, T., Goodman, R., & Meltzer, H. (2003). The British child and adolescent mental health survey 1999: The prevalence of DSM IV disorders. *Journal of the American Academy of Child and Adolescent. Psychiatry, 42,* 1203-1211.

Frazier, J. A., Biederman, J., Bellordre, C. A., Garfield, S. B., Geller, D. A., Coffey, B. J., et al. (2001). Should the diagnosis of Attention Deficit/Hyperactivity Disorder be considered in children with Pervasive Developmental Disorder? *Journal of Attention Disorders, 4*, 203-211.

Freeman, R. D., Fast, D. K., Burd, L., Kerbeshian, J. K., Robertson, M. M., & Sandor, P. (2000). An international perspective on Tourette syndrome: Selected findings from 3500 individuals in 22 countries. *Developmental Medicine and Child Neurology, 42*, 436-477.

Gerralda, M. E. (1984). Hallucinations in children with conduct and emotional disorders, I: The clinical phenomena. *Psychological Medicine, 14*, 589-596.

Goldstein, S. & Schweback, A. J. (2002). Does ADHD occur with pervasive developmental disorder? *ADHD Report, 10*(6), 1-5.

Greenspan, S. & Granfield, J. M. (1992). Reconsidering the construct of mental retardation: Implications of a model of social competence. *American Journal of Mental Retardation, 96*, 442-453.

Harris, J. C. (2001). Psychiatric disorders in mentally retarded persons. In G.O. Gabbard (Ed.), *Treatments of Psychiatric disorders* (3rd ed., pp. 75-107). Washington, DC: American Psychiatric Publishing, Inc.

Hodapp, R. M. & Dykens, E. M. (2001). Strengthening behavioral research on genetic mental retardation syndromes. *American Journal in Mental Retardation, 106*, 4-15.

Hollander, E. (1993). Introduction. In E. Hollander (Ed.), *Obsessive-Compulsive Related Disorders* (pp. 1-16). Washington, DC: American Psychiatric Press Inc.

Hudziak, J. J. (2001). The role of phenotypes (diagnoses) in genetic studies of attention-deficit/hyperactivity disorder and related child psychopathology. In R. D. Todd (Ed.), *Child and Adolescent Psychiatric Clinics of North America* Vol. 10. *Genetic Contributions to Early – Onset Psychopathology* (pp. 279-298). Philadelphia: W. B. Saunders Co.

Jan, J. E., Freeman, R. D., & Fast, D. K. (1999). Melatonin treatment of sleep-wake cycle disorders in children and adolescents. *Developmental Medicine and Child Neurology, 41*, 491-500.

Jankovic, J. (2001). Tourette's syndrome. *New England Journal of Medicine, 345*, 1184-1192.

Kado, S. & Takagi, R., (1996). Biological aspects. In S. Sandbag (Ed.), *Hyperactivity disorders of childhood* (pp. 246-279). New York: Cambridge University Press.

Kastner, T., Friedman, D. L., Plummer, A. T., Ruiz, M. Q., & Henning, D. (1990). Valproic acid for the treatment of children with mental retardation and mood symptomatology. *Pediatrics, 86*, 467-472.

King, B. H., De Antonia, C., McCracken, J. T., Forness, S. R., & Ackerland, V. (1994). Psychiatric consultation in severe and profound mental retardation. *American Journal of Psychiatry, 151*, 1802-1808.

King, B. H., State, M. W., Shah, B., Davanzo, P., & Dykens, E. (1997). Mental retardation: A review of the past 10 years. Part I. *Journal of the American Academy of Child and Adolescent Psychiatry, 36*, 1656-1663.

Klin, A., & Volkmar, F. R., (2002). Asperger syndrome: Diagnosis and external validity. In A. Klin & F. R. Volkmar (Eds.), *Child and adolescent clinics of North America* Vol. 12: *Asperger Syndrome* (pp. 1-14). Philadelphia: W. B. Saunders Co.

Kristensen, H. (2002). Selective mutism and comorbidity with developmental disorder/delay, anxiety disorder, and elimination disorder. *Journal of the American Academy of Child and Adolescent Psychiatry, 39*, 249-256.

Lacey, E. P. (1993). Phenomenology of pica. In J. L. Woolston (Ed.), *Child and adolescent clinics of North America: Eating and growth disorders* (pp. 75-91). Philadelphia: W. B. Saunders Co.

Leckman, J. F., Walker, D. E., Goodman, W. K., Pauls, D. L., & Cohen, D. J. (1994). "Just right" perceptions associated with compulsive behavior in Tourette's syndrome. *American Journal of Psychiatry, 151*, 675-680.

Lee, P., Friedlander, R., & Donnelly, C. (1998). Childhood schizophrenia in the developmentally disabled. *The NADD Bulletin, 1*, 7-11.

Lewinsoh, P. M., Klein, D. N., & Seeley, J. R. (1995) Bipolar disorders in a community sample of older adolescents: Prevalence phenomenology, comorbidity, and course. *Journal of the American Academy of Child and Adolescent Psychiatry, 34*, 454-463.

Loeber, R., Burke, J. D., Lahey, B. B., Winters, A., & Zera, M. (2000). Oppositional defiant and conduct disorder: A review of the past 10 years, Part 1. *Journal of the American Academy of Child and Adolescent Psychiatry, 39*, 1468-1484.

Malhotra, S. & Gupta, N. (1999). Childhood disintegrative disorder. *Journal of Autism and Developmental Disorders, 29*, 491-498.

Manjiviona, J., & Prior, M. (1999). Neuropsychological profiles of children with Asperger syndrome and autism. *Autism, 3*, 327-356.

McCraken, J. T. & Diamond, R. P. (1998). Case study: Bipolar disorder in mentally retarded adolescents. *Journal of the American Academy of Child and Adolescent Psychiatry, 27*, 494-499.

McGee, R., Williams, S., & Poulton, R. (2000). Hallucinations in nonpsychotic children. *Journal of the American Academy of Child and Adolescent Psychiatry, 31*, 12-13 (letter).

Mesibov, G. B., Adams, L. W. & Klinger, L. G., (1997). *Autism: Understanding the Disorder* (p. 34). New York: Plenum Press.

Mester, C. S. & Loschen, E. L., (1997). Comprehensive treatment approaches to anxiety disorders. *The NADD Newsletter, 14*, 65-68.

Moreau, C. & Zisook, S. (2002). Rationale for a posttraumatic stress spectrum disorder. In J. D. Maser & H. S. Akiskal (Eds.), *The psychiatric clinics of North America* Vol. 25: *Spectrum concepts in major mental disorders* (pp. 775-790). Philadelphia.

Nezu, C. M. & Nezu, A. M., (1994). Outpatient psychotherapy for adults with mental retardation and concomitant psychopathology: Research and clinical imperatives. *Journal of Consulting and Clinical Psychology, 62*, 34-42.

Ozonoff, S., & Rogers, S. J., (2003) From Kanner to the millennium. In S. Ozonoff, S. J. Rogers, & R. L. Hendren (Eds.), *Autism spectrum disorders: A research review for practitioners* (p. 3-36). Washington, DC: American Psychiatric Publishing, Inc.

Ozonoff, S., Rogers, S. J., & Hendren, R. L. (Eds.) (2003). *Autism spectrum disorders: A research review for practitioners.* Washington, DC: American Psychiatric Publishing, Inc.

Ozonoff, S., South, M., & Miller, J. N., (2000). DSM-IV defined Asperger syndrome: Cognitive, behavioral and early history differentiation from high-functioning autism. *Autism, 4*, 29-46.

Pavuluri, M. N., Naylor, M.W., & Janicak, P.G. (2002). Recognition and treatment of pediatric bipolar disorder. *Contemporary Psychiatry, 1*(1), 1-10.

Pawlarcyzk, D. & Beckwith, B. E., (1987). Depressive symptoms displayed by persons with mental retardation: A review. *Mental Retardation, 25*, 325-330.

Pearson, D. A., Lachar, D., Loveland, K. A., Santos, C. W., Faria, L. P. Azzam, P. N., et al. (2000). Patterns of behavioral adjustment and maladjustment in mental retardation: Comparison of children with and without ADHD. *American Journal on Mental Retardation, 105*, 236-251.

Perry, B. D. & Polland, R., (1998). Homeostasis, stress, trauma, and adaptation: A neurodevelopmental view of childhood trauma. In B. Pfefferbaum (Ed.), *Child and adolescent clinics of North America* Vol. 7: *Stress in children* (pp. 33-52). Philadelphia: W. B. Saunders Co.

Pfefferbaum, B. & Allen, J. R., (1998). Stress in children exposed to violence: Reenactment and rage. In B. Pfefferbaum (Ed.), *Child and adolescent clinics of North America* Vol. 7: *Stress in children* (pp. 121-136). Philadelphia: W. B. Saunders Co.

Phillips, K. A. (2002). The obsessive-compulsive spectrums. In J. D. Maser & H. S. Akiskal (Eds.), *The psychiatric clinics of North America* Vol. 25: *Spectrum concepts in major mental disorders* (pp. 791-809). Philadelphia: W. B. Saunders Co.

Piazza, C. C., Fisher, W. W., & Kahng, S. W. (1996). Sleep patterns in children and young adults with mental retardation and severe behavior disorders. *Developmental Medicine and Child Neurology, 38*, 335-344.

Pliszka, S. R., Carlson, C. L., & Swanson, J. M., (1999). Epilogue: Future directions in research and treatment. In S. R. Pliszka, C. L. Carlson, & J. M. Swanson, (Eds.), *ADHD with comorbid disorders clinical assessment and management* (pp. 261-270). New York: The Guilford Press.

Poindexter, A.R. (1998). Sleep disorders in persons with mental retardation – a significant factor in many behavioral/psychiatric problems? *NADD Bulletin, 1*, 89-91.

Popper, C. W., Gammon, G. D., West, S. A., & Bailey, C. E., (2003). Disorders usually first diagnosed in infancy, childhood, or adolescence. In R. E. Hales & S. C. Yudofsky (Eds.), *The American psychiatric publishing textbook of clinical psychiatry* (pp. 833-976). Washington, DC: American Psychiatric Publishing, Inc.

Quine, L. (1991). Sleep problems in children with mental handicap. *Journal of Mental Deficiency Research, 35*, 269-290.

Reba, R. C. (1993). PET and SPECT: Opportunities and challenges for psychiatry. *Journal of Clinical Psychiatry, 54*(Suppl.) 26-32.

Rena, L. & El-Mallakh, R. (1997). Triplet repeat gene sequences in neuropsychiatric diseases. *Harvard Review of Psychiatry, 5*, 66-74.

Robertson, M. M. (1992). Self-injurious behavior and Tourette syndrome. *Advances in Neurology, 58*, 105-114.

Rosenn, D. W. (1999). What is Asperger's disorder? *The Harvard Mental Health Letter, 16*(4), 8.

Russell, A. T., Bott, L., & Sammons, C. (1989). The phenomenology of schizophrenia occurring in childhood. *Journal of the American Academy of Child and Adolescent Psychiatry, 28*, 399-407.

Rutter, M., Tizard, J., Yule, W., Graham, P., & Whitmore, K. (1976). Research report: Isle of Wight studies, 1964-74. *Psychological Medicine, 6,* 313-332.

Ryan, R. M., (1996[a]). Beam up the universal translator: Interpretation of DSM-IV for persons who use little or no spoken language. In R. M. Ryan, *Handbook of mental health care for persons with Developmental Disabilities* (pp. 179-192). Evergreen, CO: S & B Publishing.

Ryan, R. M., (1996[b]). Teach me a new language: Recognizing psychosis in people who do not speak. In R. M. Ryan, *Handbook of mental health care for persons with Developmental Disabilities* (pp. 67-78). Evergreen, CO: S & B Publishing.

Salimpoor, V. N. (2003). Advances in neuroimaging of autistic spectrum disorder and other Developmental Disabilities. *The NADD Bulletin, 6,* 112-115.

Scheeringa, M. S., Zeanah, C. H., Drell, M. J., & Larrieu, J. A. (1995). Two approaches to the diagnosis of posttraumatic stress disorder in infancy and early childhood. *Journal of the American Academy of Child and Adolescent Psychiatry, 34,* 191-200.

Schreier, H. A. (1999). Hallucinations in nonpsychotic children: More common than we think? *Journal of the American Academy of Child and Adolescent Psychiatry, 38,* 623-625.

Semper, T. F., & McClellan, J. M. (2003). The psychotic child. In M. Lewis (Ed.), *Child and Adolescent Psychiatric Clinics of North America* Vol. 12*: Psychiatric Emergencies* (pp. 679-691). Philadelphia: W. B. Saunders Co.

Sigman, M., Dissanayake, C., Arbelle, S., & Ruskin, E. (1997). Cognition and emotion in children and adolescents with autism. In D. J. Cohen & F. R. Volkmar (Eds.), *Handbook of autism and pervasive Developmental Disorders* (pp. 248-265). New York: John Wiley & Sons, Inc.

Simpson, J. A. (1999). Attachment theory in modern evolutionary perspective. In J. Cassidy & P. R. Shaver (Eds.), *Handbook of attachment: Theory, research, and clinical applications* (pp. 115-140). New York: The Guilford Press.

Siperstein, G. H., Leffert, J. S., & Wenz-Gross, M. (1997). The quality of friendships between children with and without learning problems. *American Journal of Mental Retardation, 102,* 111-125.

Smith, M. B. (2003). Behavioral forms of stress management for individuals with Asperger syndrome. In A. Klin & F. R. Volkmar (Eds.), *Child and adolescent psychiatric clinics of North America* Vol. 12*: Asperger Syndrome* (pp. 123-142). Philadelphia: W. B. Saunders Co.

Sovner, R. (1986). Limiting factors in the use of DSM-III criteria with mentally ill/mentally retarded persons. *Psychopharmacology Bulletin, 22,* 1055-1059.

Sovner, R., & Hurley, A. (1986). Managing aggressive behavior: A psychiatric approach. *Psychiatric Aspects of Mental Retardation, 5,* 16-21.

Sporn, A., & Rapoport, J. L., (2001). Childhood onset schizophrenia. *Child & Adolescent Psychopharmacology News, 6*(2), 1-6.

Steffenburg, S. Gillberg, C., & Steffenburg, U. (1996). Psychiatric disorders in children and adolescents with mental retardation and active epilepsy. *Archives of Neurology, 53,* 904-912.

Stromme, P., & Diseth, T. H. (2000). Prevalence of psychiatric diagnosis in children with mental retardation: Data from a population-based study. *Developmental Medicine and Child Neurology, 42*, 266-270.

Sutcliffe, J. S., & Nurmi, E. L. (2003). Genetics of childhood disorders: XLVII. Autism, part 6: Duplication and inherited susceptibility of chromosome 15q11-q13 genes in autism. *Journal of the American Academy of Child and Adolescent Psychiatry, 42*, 253-256.

Sverd, J., Dubey, D. R., Schweitzer, R., & Ninan, R. (2003). Pervasive developmental disorders among children and adolescents attending psychiatric day treatment. *Psychiatric Services, 54*, 1519-1525.

Szymanski, L. S., King, B., Goldberg, B., Reid, A., Tonge, B., & Cain, N. (1998). Diagnosis of mental disorders in people with mental retardation. In S. Reiss & M. G. Aman (Eds.), *Psychotropic medication Developmental Disabilities: The international consensus handbook* (pp. 3-18). Columbus, OH: The Ohio State University Nisonger Center.

Thompson, R. A., (1999). Early attachment and later development. In R. Cassidy & P. R. Shaver (Eds.), *Handbook of attachment: Theory, research, and clinical applications* (pp. 265-286). New York: The Guilford Press.

Tonge, B. J. (1999). Psychopathology of children with developmental disabilities. In N. Bouras (Ed.), *Psychiatric and behavioral disorders in Developmental Disabilities and Mental Retardation* (pp. 157-174). New York: Cambridge University Press.

Tonge, B. J., Einfeld, S. L., Krupinski, J., Mackenzie, A., McLaughlin, M., Florio, T., & Nunn, R.J. (1996). The use of factor analysis for ascertaining patterns of psychopathology in children with intellectual disability. *Journal of Intellectual Disability Research, 40*, 198-207.

Tsi, L.Y. (1994). Rett syndrome. In F. R. Volkmar (Ed.), *Child and adolescent psychiatric clinics of North America* Vol. 3: *Psychoses and pervasive Developmental Disorder* (pp. 105-118). Philadelphia: W. B. Saunders Co.

Tsiouris, J. A. (2001). Diagnosis of depression in people with severe/profound intellectual disability. *Journal of Intellectual Disability Research, 45*, 115-120.

Ulloa, R. E., Birmaher, B., Axelson, D., Williamson, D. E., Brent, D. A., Ryan, N. D., et al. (2000). Psychosis in a pediatric mood and anxiety disorders clinic: Phenomenology and correlates. *Journal of the American Academy of Child and Adolescent Psychiatry, 39*, 337-345.

Vanstraelen, M. & Tyrer, S. P. (1999). Rapid cycling bipolar affective disorder in people with intellectual disability: A systematic review. *Journal of Intellectual Disability Research, 43*, 349-359.

Veenstra-Vanderweele, J. & Cook, E. H. (2003). Genetics of childhood disorders: XLVI. Autism; part 5: Genetics of autism. *Journal of the American Academy of Child and Adolescent Psychiatry, 42*, 116-118.

Volkmar, F. R. & Dykens, E. (2002). Mental retardation. In M. Rutter & E. Taylor (Eds.), *Child and adolescent psychiatry* (pp. 697-710). Malden, MA: Blackwell Science Inc.

Volkmar, F. R. & Klin, A. (2000). Diagnostic issues in Asperger syndrome. In A. Klin, F. R. Volkmar, & S. S. Sparrow (Eds.), *Asperger Syndrome* (pp. 25-71). New York: The Guilford Press.

Volkmar, F. R., Klin, A., & Cohen, D. J. (1997). Diagnosis and classification of autism and related conditions: Consensus and issues. In D. J. Cohen & F. R. Volkmar (Eds.), *Handbook of autism and pervasive Developmental Disorders* (pp. 5-40). New York: John Wiley & Sons, Inc.

Volkmar, F. R., Klin, A., Marans, W., & Cohen, D. J. (1997). Childhood disintegrative disorder. In D. J. Cohen & F. R. Volkmar (Eds.), *Handbook of autism and pervasive Developmental Disorders* (2nd ed., pp. 47-59). New York: John Wiley & Sons.

Volkmar, F. R. & Rutter, M. (1995). Childhood disintegrative disorder: Results of the DSM-IV autism field trial. *Journal of the American Academy of Child and Adolescent Psychiatry, 34*, 1092-1095.

Walkup, J. T., Scahill, L. D., & Riddle, M. A. (1995). Disruptive behavior, hyperactivity, and learning disabilities in children with Tourette's syndrome. *Advances in Neurology, 65*, 259-272.

Weisz, J. R. (1990). Cultural-familial mental retardation: A developmental perspective on cognitive performance and "helpless" behavior. In R. M. Hodapp, J. A. Burack, & E. Zigler (Eds.), *Issues in the Developmental Approach to Mental Retardation* (pp. 137-168). New York: Cambridge University Press.

Wing, L. (1981). Asperger's syndrome: A clinical account. *Psychological Medicine, 11*, 115-130.

Wing, L. (1991). The relationship between Asperger's syndrome and Kanner's autism. In U. Frith (Ed.), *Autism and Asperger syndrome* (pp. 93-121). New York: Cambridge University Press.

Wolke, D., Meyer, R., Ohrt, B., & Riegel, K. (1995). Comorbidity of crying and feeding problems with sleeping problems in infancy: Concurrent and predictive associations. *Early Development and Parenting, 4*, 1-17.

World Health Organization (WHO), (1992). *The ICD-10 classification of mental and behavioral disorders clinical descriptions and diagnostic guidelines.* Geneva, Switzerland: World Health Organization.

Zeanah, C. H. & Boris, N. W. (2000). Disturbances and disorders of attachment in early childhood. In C. H. Zeanah (Ed.), *Handbook of infant mental health,* (2nd ed., pp. 353-368). New York: The Guilford Press.

Zohar, A. H., Pauls, D. L. Ratzoni, G., Apter, A., Dycian, A., Binder, M., et al. (1997). Obsessive-compulsive disorder with and without tics in an epidemiological sample of adolescents. *American Journal of Psychiatry, 154*, 274-276.

5

Prevalence of Behavioral Disturbance

John W. Jacobson

INTRODUCTION

This chapter presents information about the prevalence of a wide variety of behavior disturbances: how prevalence differs with age and level of intellectual functioning; the co-occurrence of specific behaviors with mental disorders, findings with respect to the topology of several behaviors; the relative prevalence of aggression, self-injury, and destructive behavior, and behaviors associated with referral for services. A behavior disturbance is defined as behaviors that are socially unacceptable, interfere with social interaction, and differ from social expectations for conduct (Fraser & Nolan, 1994). In common clinical usage the term behavioral disturbance is largely synonymous with a number of other terms, including behavior disorders, maladaptive behaviors, problem behaviors, or behavior problems (Cooper, 1998; Lowe & Felce, 1995). Such behaviors may or may not co-occur with a diagnosed mental disorder. Specific behavioral disturbances constitute a clinically significant complicating factor when they co-occur with mental disorders and require significant treatment focus when such co-occurrence is not evident, because of the extent to which such behavioral disturbances may interfere with societal participation.

BEHAVIOR DISORDERS AND MENTAL DISORDERS

Pathways by which behaviors and mental disorders may be related in people with ID include:
- Familial, based upon developmental or social history;
- An atypical presentation of a mental disorder;
- A secondary feature of a mental disorder, or
- Behaviors triggered by a mental disorder but maintained by environmental factors (Emerson, Moss, & Kiernan, 1999).

Mental disorders cannot be assumed to always cause behavioral disturbances when they co-occur. Under some circumstances, it may not be possible to determine the specific cause or causes of a behavioral disturbance, although it may be possible to identify factors that maintain or influence the occurrence of the behavior. There are behavioral phenotypes in which characteristic behaviors and patterns of behaviors are associated with the presence of genotypic disorders or conditions (Dykens, 2000). Different patterns of self-injury or other behavioral disturbances are associated with some genetic syndromes (e.g., Down syndrome, Fragile X syndrome, Prader-Willi syndrome, Smith-Magenis syndrome, Williams syndrome, and Cri du Chat syndrome). Syndromes such as these may co-occur with mental disorders; in such instances causal linkages may not be evident.

PREVALENCE OF SPECIFIC BEHAVIOR DISORDERS

Research to determine the prevalence of specific behavioral disturbances may be influenced by a number of factors including:
- Variation in the definitions of target behaviors (the behavior actually measured);
- Differences among the characteristics of participants (e.g., people in certain residential settings, as opposed to all people with ID), and
- Variation in methods used to gather information (e.g., population-based groups or groups that may or may not be representative of the larger population of people with ID).

Table 5.1 shows the percentages of a large cohort of New Yorkers with ID in six age groups, and separately with mental disorders and ID, for whom a wide range of specific behavior disorders are reported to occur in the Developmental Disabilities Information System database (Janicki & Jacobson, 1982 to 1988). Such databases are rare. When available and well-defined, they can shed useful light on epidemiological questions such as prevalence rates. The proportion of people with no reported behavioral disturbance is greatest among preschoolers, school age children, and people age 75 years or older. Most behaviors occur at their highest rates among adults between ages 22 and 59 years. Exceptions to this pattern are hyperactivity or stereotypic movements, which are more frequent among school-age children, and delusions, hallucinations, or disorientation as well as irritability, depression, or mood changes, which are reported to occur at higher levels among older people. Individuals with mental disorders and ID are far more likely to have a co-occurring behavioral disturbance than are people with ID alone.

Table 5.2 shows data from a study of 519 Australian children with ID, aged from birth to 18 years, using the Developmental Behavior Checklist (DBC) (Einfeld & Tonge, 1995); 33% were classified with mild ID, the remainder with severe ID (Sherrard & Tonge, 1997). These findings suggest that some specific behaviors or behavioral descriptors that pose risk for injury (the focus of their study) may diminish from earlier to later childhood. Most of these behaviors remain relatively common through age 13 to 18 years. Data in this table are arranged according to the DBC factor subscales of Self-absorbed, Disruptive, and Antisocial.

Jacobson (1982) reported behavior disorder prevalence for children (N=1,627 with mild ID, 7,101 with severe ID) and adults (N=4,163 with mild ID, 17,686 with severe ID) in New York State (similar data on population samples have been presented by Einfeld & Tonge, 1996; Emerson et al., 2001; Joyce, Ditchfield, & Harris, 2001; Lakin, Bruininks, Chen, Hill, & Anderson, 1993). For children and adults: disorientation, suicide threats or attempts, assault, property destruction, self-injury, genital display, disrobing, stereotypy, handling of bodily wastes, and pica occurred less frequently among people with mild ID than with severe ID, regardless of age. Other behaviors, including depression, irritability, fire-setting or attempts, verbal abuse to others, blaming others, and substance abuse occurred more frequently among both children and adults with mild ID. Among children with mild ID, the most frequent specific behaviors included temper tantrums and resisting supervision, while among adults, lack of responsiveness and verbal abuse were most frequent. Among children with severe ID, temper tantrums, lack of responsiveness, assault, self-injury, and hyperactivity were most common, and among adults, assault, lack of responsiveness, and self-injury were most frequent.

TABLE 5.1
Prevalence of Behavior Disorders among Individuals with Mild ID (Percents of Cases)

	Age Group in Years (N=60,847)						
	Mental disorders and ID and Non-Mental disorders and ID Combined						Mental disorders and ID only
	<5	5-21	22-39	40-59	60-74	>74	(All Ages)
Behavioral Category							
None	79	47	33	31	37	50	12
Assault/Sexual Behavior	2	10	15	13	10	5	22
Disrobing	0	1	3	3	2	9	3
Self-Injury/Suicide Attempt	2	7	11	9	4	2	13
Delusions/Hallucinations/Disorientation	1	4	5	8	11	13	16
Perseveration/Echolalia	2	5	5	5	4	3	8
Irritibility/Depression/Mood Changes	2	9	15	19	2	16	33
Pica/Handles Bodily Wastes	1	2	4	4	3	3	3
Hyperactivity/Stereotypic Movements	5	16	13	10	5	2	16
Tantrums/Verbal Abuse/Resists Treatment	17	25	29	34	33	22	30
Inappropriate Affect/Socially Unresponsive	5	17	20	20	17	15	31
Other	4	19	28	25	20	12	32

TABLE 5.2
Percents of Selected Behavioral Characteristics Posing Risk Factors for Injury

Scales and Items	Age in Years (N)		
	<9 (152)	9-12 (152)	13-18 (260)
Self-Absorbed			
Poor sense of danger	74	68	53
Chews or mouths objects or body parts	45	26	31
Deliberately runs away	42	26	21
Eats non-food items	19	17	10
Hits self or bites self	29	29	19.1
Bangs head	15	14	14
Disruptive			
Impulsive; acts before thinking	57	50	50
Has temper tantrums	60	54	59
Talks about suicide	2	3	7
Antisocial			
Lights fires	3	7	5
Unclassified			
Scratches or picks his/her skin	21	26	30
Smells, tastes, or licks objects	29	29	20
Gorges food (will do anything to get food)	15	16	13

PHARMACOLOGICAL TREATMENT OF SPECIFIC BEHAVIORAL DISTURBANCES

Table 5.3 shows the rate at which specific behaviors were treated using psychotropic medication. These data provide some indication of the behaviors that are likely to be present when people with ID or people with mental disorders and ID are prescribed these types of medications. They should not be interpreted to indicate that particular behaviors are the primary target symptoms when these medications are prescribed.

Overall, adults with mental disorders and ID present more behavior disorders than do people with ID alone. While prevalence is not shown in Table 5.3, the data suggests that suicide threats or attempts, delusions or hallucinations, mood changes, preservation, depression, fire-setting or attempts, irritability, inappropriate affect, coercive sexual behavior, and substance abuse occur at higher rates among adults with mental disorders and ID. This could be expected, as many of these behaviors are consistent with the criteria for some mental disorders. However, some behavioral disturbances also occur at fairly similar rates for adults with ID and those with mental disorders and ID, including self-injurious behavior, genital display, handling wastes, pica, temper tantrums, stereotypic behavior, and property theft.

TABLE 5.3
Psychotropic Medication Frequency (Percents) among Individuals with ID*

Behavioral Diagnosis	Mental disorders and ID (3,341)	No Mental disorder and ID (31,666)
Disrobing	86	53
Suicide threats or attempts	80	43
Physical assault	79	56
Property destruction	79	51
Delusions/hallucinations	77	51
Self-injurious behavior	76	52
Genital display	73	40
Mood changes	73	42
Handles wastes	72	49
Pica	70	41
Perseveration	68	39
Depression	68	34
Verbally abusive	67	32
Wanders/roams	67	33
Temper tantrums	67	32
Fire-setting or attempts	67	44
Irritability	66	28
Echolalia	65	35
Hyperactivity	65	17
Disorientation	64	39
Stereotyped behaviors	62	27
Inappropriate affect	62	38
Coercive sexual behavior	61	28
Resists supervision	31	27
Interpersonal unresponsive	25	33
Property theft	30	28
Substance abuse	17	37
Blames others	19	34

*Unpublished data from the population studied by Jacobson (1988).

For both people with ID and those with mental disorders and ID, physical assault, property destruction, and self-injury are among the specific behavioral disturbances most often associated with medication as a treatment component. Research on antipsychotic medication effects in people with ID has recently been reviewed by Brylewski & Dugan (1999), and contemporary treatment guidelines are available (Reiss & Aman, 1998; Rush & Frances, 2000). Findings with regard to benefits of psychotropic medications upon behavioral disturbances not co-occurring with mental disorders have often been discouraging, with interpretation of findings limited by small sample sizes. As Sovner & Hurley (1999) have noted, "for many [mental] conditions, drug therapy is the primary treatment of choice, and for some conditions (such as manic states), drug therapy is the only active treatment." However, some behaviors such as self-injury and aggression, which may not be derivative of a mental disorder, are "too nonspecific to be considered as direct targets for drug therapy." Medication has not been well-supported as the primary treatment for these behaviors when they do not represent atypical presentations or secondary features of a mental disorder or are not triggered primarily by a mental disorder.

BEHAVIORAL TRIAD: AGGRESSION, SELF-INJURY, AND DESTRUCTIVE BEHAVIOR

Topology of Behavior Disorders

Aggression (upon others), self-injury (aggression toward self), and destructive behaviors (aggression toward or involving objects) are among the most severe behavioral disturbances that occur among people with ID. Recent research has found that the most frequent forms of aggressive behavior among adults with ID are grabbing, hitting, self-injury, throwing objects, scratching, or kicking (Joyce, Ditchfield & Harris, 2001). The most common forms of non-aggressive behavior within this same sample are refusal to participate in activities, making loud noises, shouting or swearing, withdrawing from others, or slamming doors. Other research has also reported that the most common forms of aggression among children and adults with ID are hitting others with hands, verbal aggression, hitting others with objects, and meanness or cruelty (Emerson et al., 2001). The most frequent forms of self-injury are hitting one's head or body against self or objects, or biting oneself. Other common problem behaviors that have been noted include generalized noncompliance, temper tantrums, repetitive pestering, and screaming.

Prevalence of a Triad

Jacobson & Ackerman (1993) estimated the prevalence of aggression, self-injury, and destructive behavior in adults with ID using the Developmental Disabilities Profile described earlier. The population prevalence of these three behaviors has not been estimated elsewhere. Aggression occurred most frequently, followed by destructive behavior, and self-injury. Table 5.4 also shows these prevalence rates, by intellectual level, for each of the triad of behaviors, with 2.4% to 4.7% of adults with mild ID and from 11.1% to 14.4% of adults with severe ID evidencing each behavior, and 0.73% and 3.3%, respectively manifesting all three behaviors.

TABLE 5.4
Prevalence of Aggression, Self-injury and Destructive Behavior

Behavior	Percent of Cases*	
	Mild ID	Severe ID
Aggression	5	14
Self-injury	3	12
Destructive behavior	2	11
One of three	4	14
Two of three	1	6
Three of three	1	3

Treatment of the Triad

Sometimes people with ID receive antipsychotic medication in the course of treatment for reasons other than the triad of behavioral disturbances. However, these rates increase substantially if one or more of these three behavior disorders are present (Jacobson, 1993). Generally, living at home with family is consistently associated with the minimum rates of receipt of either antipsychotic medication or behavior intervention for people with one or more of these three behavior disorders (Jacobson 1992). Adults with any of these behavior disorders, moreover, and perhaps contrary to conventional wisdom, are more likely to receive behavior intervention services than treatment with antipsychotic medications for these behavioral disturbances (Jacobson 1993). Research findings for behavior intervention as the primary treatment for this triad have been summarized most comprehensively by the National Institute of Health (1989), and treatment guidelines have been presented by Rush & Frances (2000).

REFERRAL FOR SERVICES

Several research reports have identified factors associated with referral of people with ID for mental health or crisis intervention services, based on approximately 250 to 400 referrals (Davidson et al., 1995; Edelstein & Glenwick, 1997; Shoham-Vardi, Davidson, & Cain, 1996). Primary referral reasons have included externalizing behavior (including physical or verbal aggression, property destruction, or noncompliance); internal behavior (depressive symptoms including dysphoric mood, frequent crying, hopelessness, mood swings); social deficits (including annoying others, lack of friends, poor social skills), and psychotic symptoms (including delusions, hallucinations, inappropriate affect, peculiar behaviors). Referrals related to psychosexual dysfunction and substance abuse seem to be comparatively rare.

One of the most common referral reasons involves aggression, including assault or property destruction, followed closely by noncompliance, including oppositional behavior or refusal to participate in services or perform daily tasks. First referral for aggression or self-injury has been reported to be a predictor of re-referral, indicating that service agencies may encounter particular difficulty in implementing prescribed behavioral treatments or maintaining fidelity of treatment practices when these problems are present. These patterns of re-referral are consistent with the findings from a clinic sample (Shoham-Vardi et al., 1996) that there were typically no changes in ratings of behavior consistent with the original behavioral disturbance over a four-year period, for between 70% and 85% of the participants, with approximately equal proportions of the others showing improvement or deterioration of behavior (Tonge & Einfeld, 2000).

SUMMARY

This chapter indicates that estimating the prevalence of specific behavior disorders among persons with ID may be very difficult. The findings from one study often cannot be combined or compared with those from others because of differences in the samples used. Sometimes this is a matter of evident differences in samples, such as differences in how samples are divided into age or ability groups. In other instances, there are meaningful differences in how data about behavioral disturbances are defined, or disorders are identified that prevent reconciliation of findings from one study with another. These issues hinder prevalence estimates of specific behavior disorders.

Nonetheless, there are some generalities that can be asserted with some confidence:

- People with mental disorders and mild ID tend to manifest a wide range of specific behavioral disturbances at higher rates than their peers with mild ID alone. Although there may be a causal link between the presence of a mental disorder and a specific behavioral disturbance, there is little evidence that this can be assumed in the individual case and research has not fully addressed this issue;

- Specific behavioral disturbances can be persistent, both as reported based on re-referral and follow-up, and as suggested by age group patterns in which the occurrence of some behavioral disturbances increase from youth into adulthood;

- Clinically significant proportions of people served in the ID sector evidence one or more behaviors, including aggression, self-injury, or property destruction; all of these typically compromise personal safety or jeopardize health while posing risk of admission to restrictive settings and often stimulating crisis or mental-health-service referral;

- Although presence of mental disorder symptoms is commonly associated with prescription treatment with psychoactive medication, so is presence of behavior disturbances that may or may not be associated with a mental disorder in the individual case. At the same time, research findings indicate that treatment with medication typically occurs conjointly with behavioral treatment, and

- Existing prevalence data indicate that the occurrence of mental disorders, behavioral disturbances, and co-occurring mental and behavioral disturbances differs within the population of people with ID based on the degree of ID. The extent to which this is an artifact of available diagnostic skills or a reflection of developmental and other personal factors, is presently unknown.

Despite the broad nature of the conclusions that can currently be drawn regarding behavioral disturbances and the limited understanding that we have of their developmental course, it is apparent that they are sufficiently prevalent to stimulate substantial numbers of referrals for care. As noted elsewhere in this book (Chapter 10), there is a significant need for specialized expertise in local service systems to alleviate the impact of behavioral disturbances and diminish their persistence. Because of the long-standing focus on habilitative and supportive services, diminished focus on treatment, and increased emphasis on supports in community developmental services, availability of experts in ID and mental disorders to serve people with co-existing mental and behavioral disturbances remains limited. In many rural areas, specialized practitioners may be unavailable, and in urban areas, demands or referrals for services still may outstrip the capacity of practitioners and programs to provide specialized care.

As the data presented in this chapter has indicated, many of the behavioral disturbances occurring among people with ID are threatening to their own health and safety, pose risk for injury, or can engender fear or social ostracism by others. In many cases, to effectively assure that caregivers can provide the components of intervention necessary for overall therapeutic success, community clinicians may have to extend their services to include coaching, training, and guidance for caregivers as well as direct therapeutic intervention for the person with ID.

REFERENCES

Brylewski, J. & Duggan, L. (1999). Review: Antipsychotic medication for challenging behavior in people with intellectual disability: A systematic review of randomized controlled trials. *Journal of Intellectual Disability Research, 43,* 360-371.

Cooper, S. A. (1998). Behaviour disorders in adults with learning disabilities: Effect of age and differentiation from other psychiatric disorders. *Irish Journal of Psychological Medicine, 15,* 13-18.

Davidson, P. W., Cain, N. N., Sloane-Reeves, J. E., Giesow, V. W., Quijano, L. E., Van Heynigen, J., & Shoham, I. (1995). Crisis intervention for community-based individuals with developmental disabilities and behavioral and psychiatric disorders. *Intellectual Disabilities, 33,* 21-30.

Dykens, E. M. (2000). Annotation: Psychopathology in children with intellectual disability. *Journal of Child Psychology and Psychiatry, 41,* 407-417.

Edelstein, T. M. & Glenwick, D. S. (1997). Referral reasons for psychological services for adults with Intellectual Disabilities. *Research in Developmental Disabilities, 18,* 45-59.

Einfeld, S. L. & Tonge, B. J. (1995). The Developmental Behavior Checklist: The development and validation of an instrument to assess behavioral and emotional disturbance in children and adolescents with Intellectual Disabilities. *Journal of Autism & Development, 25*(2) 81-104.

Einfeld, S. L. & Tonge, J. (1996). Population prevalence of psychopathology in children and adolescents with intellectual disability: II. Epidemiological findings. *Journal of Intellectual Disability Research, 40,* 99-109.

Emerson, E., Kiernan, C., Alborz, A., Reeves, D., Mason, H., Swarbrick, R., et al. (2001). The prevalence of Behavior Disorders: A total population study. *Research in Developmental Disabilities, 22,* 77-93.

Emerson, E., Moss, S., & Kiernan, C. (1999). The relationship between challenging behavior and psychiatric disorders in persons with severe developmental disabilities. In N. Bouras (Ed.), *Psychiatric and behavioural disorders in developmental disabilities and mental retardation* (pp. 38-48). Cambridge University Press.

Fraser, W. I., & Nolan, M. (1994). Psychiatric disorders in mental retardation. In N. Bouras (Ed.), *Mental health in mental retardation: Recent advances and practices* (pp. 79-92). Cambridge University Press.

Jacobson, J. W. (1982). Problem behavior and psychiatric impairment in a developmentally disabled population: Behavior frequency. *Applied Research in Intellectual Disabilities, 3,* 121-139.

Jacobson, J. W. (1988). Problem behavior and psychiatric impairment in a developmentally disabled population III: Psychotropic medication. *Research in Developmental Disabilities, 9,* 23-38.

Jacobson, J. W. (1992). Who is treated using restrictive behavioral procedures? *Journal of Developmental and Physical Disabilities, 4,* 99-113.

Jacobson, J. W. (1993). Public policy and the punishment of the powerless. *Child and Adolescent Mental Health Care. 3,* 7-18.

Jacobson, J. W. & Ackerman, L. J. (1993). Who is treated using restrictive procedures? A population perspective. *Research in Developmental Disabilities, 14,* 51-65.

Janicki, M. P. & Jacobson, J. W. (1982-1988). *Developmental Disabilities Information System* (DDIS): *Computer-generated summary population age-group tables.* Albany, NY: Planning Bureau, New York State Office of Mental Retardation and Developmental Disabilities.

Joyce, T., Ditchfield, H., & Harris, P. (2001). Challenging behaviour in community services. *Journal of Intellectual Disability Research, 45,* 130-138.

Lakin, K. C., Bruininks, R. H., Chen, T., Hill, B. K., & Anderson, D. (1993). Personal characteristics and competence of people with Intellectual Disabilities living in foster homes and small group homes. *American Journal on Intellectual Disabilities, 97,* 616-627.

Lowe, K. & Felce, D., (1995). The definition of challenging behavior in practice. *British Journal of Learning Disabilities, 23,*118-123.

National Institute of Health. (1989). *Treatment of destructive behaviors in persons with developmental disabilities (NIH Consensus Statement)*, Bethesda, MD.

Reiss, S. & Aman, M. G. (Eds.), (1998). *Psychotropic medications and   ies: The international consensus handbook.* Baltimore: Brookes Publishing.

Rush, A. J. & Frances, A. (Eds.), (2000). Treatment of psychiatric and behavior problems in Intellectual Disabilities. *American Journal on Intellectual Disabilities (Expert Consensus Guidelines Series), 105,* entire issue.

Sherrard, J. & Tonge, B. J. (1997). Behaviours in young people with intellectual disability: Preliminary findings and implications for injury. *Journal of Intellectual & Developmental Disability, 22*(1) 39-48.

Shoham-Vardi, I., Davidson, P. W., & Cain, N. N. (1996). Factors predicting re-referral following crisis intervention for community-based persons with developmental disabilities and behavioral and psychiatric disorders. *American Journal on Intellectual Disabilities, 101*, 109-117.

Sovner, R. & Hurley, A. D. (1999). Facts and fictions concerning psychiatric disorders in people with intellectual disabilities and developmental disabilities. In N. A. Wieseler & R. H. Hanson (Eds.), *Behavior Disorder of persons with Psychiatric Disorders and severe developmental disabilities* (pp. 89-99). Washington, DC: American Association on Intellectual Disabilities.

Tonge, B. & Einfeld, S. (2000). The trajectory of psychiatric disorders in young people with intellectual disabilities. *Australian and New Zealand Journal of Psychiatry, 34*, 80-84.

6

Autism

Caroline I. Magyar, Tristram Smith, and Jennifer Katz

INTRODUCTION

Autism, also called autistic disorder, is a chronic neurobiological condition that frequently co-occurs with developmental delay. The word autism means "absorbed in the self." The diagnosis of autism involves difficulties in social interactions (e.g., lack of reciprocity, poor eye contact), stereotyped behaviors (e.g., repeated hand-flapping), and impairments in communication (e.g., lack of speech) before age 3. Recent estimates suggest a prevalence rate of about 1 in 750 to 1 in 1,000 (Bryson & Smith, 1998), and a greater number of boys who have the disorder than girls (about 4:1). Approximately 75 percent of individuals with autism are diagnosed with intellectual disability (ID).

Individuals with dual diagnoses of autism and ID may appear to be severely withdrawn, socially awkward, or both. The social and communication problems at the core of autism restrict individuals' abilities to relate meaningfully to people and objects in their environments. Further, the significant cognitive challenges faced by individuals with both autism and ID interfere with their abilities to learn, achieve, and function autonomously.

HISTORY

Leo Kanner introduced autism to modern psychiatry in 1943. Today, autism continues to be defined based upon Kanner's original description involving (a) qualitative impairment in reciprocal social interaction; (b) qualitative impairment in verbal and nonverbal communication and in imaginative activity, and (c) markedly restricted repertoire of activities and interests (APA, 1994). Nevertheless, conceptualizations of autism have undergone two major transformations over the years.

Before the late 1960s and early 1970s, autism was widely regarded as a variant of schizophrenia. In fact, the term "autism" was derived from a classic description of schizophrenia (Bleuler, 1911/1950). However, this view became untenable when researchers demonstrated that the characteristics of autism were quite different from those of schizophrenia (Kolvin et al., 1971). Early writers considered autism to be the result of problems in the family environment. They asserted that parents, usually mothers, "caused" their children's autism because of inappropriate parenting or mental disturbances (e.g., Bettelheim, 1967). These assertions were made without empirical study and were subsequently refuted by research that showed that autism is biological rather than psychosocial in origin. By about 1970, investigators had shown that parents of children with autism were no more harsh or neglectful than other parents (DeMyer, Pontius, Norton, Barton, & Steele, 1972), and that children with autism had much more severe impairments than children with known histories of abuse (Rutter, 1972). As a result of these findings, a new consensus emerged that autism is a distinct disorder with an organic rather than psychogenic etiology.

During this period, researchers also recognized that autism was associated with delayed or atypical cognitive and language skills (Rutter, Bartak, & Newman, 1971), and that these delays could be alleviated with specialized teaching techniques (Lovaas, Berberich, Perloff, & Schaeffer, 1966). Thus, autism began to be classified as a developmental disability instead of a psychosis. Such developments led to the identification of autism as a developmental disorder warranting special education services (Education for All Handicapped Children Act, 1975). However, it remained in the standard classification system (DSM-III, American Psychiatric Association, 1980) for mental disorders. Additional changes in conceptualization occurred in the 1980s, when estimates of the prevalence of autism began to rise. The reasons for this sharp increase are currently the focus of intense investigation and debate, but one factor has clearly been important: diagnostic criteria have become more inclusive. For example, "a pervasive lack of social interaction" was a diagnostic criterion for autism in early systems (e.g., the Diagnostic and Statistical Manual of Mental Disorders, 3rd edition, or DSM-III; APA, 1980). Subsequent research suggests, however, that most individuals with autism display attachment behaviors and approach others to make requests, though not for social conversation or other reciprocal interactions (Sigman et al., 1999).

Further, research reveals large individual differences in the severity of autism. Some individuals with autism appear unaware of other people most of the time, whereas others engage and interact frequently, albeit awkwardly. Likewise, although some individuals with autism have little conventional language and communicate primarily through nonverbal means, others use age-appropriate vocabulary and syntax. Individuals with severe impairments often have a dual diagnosis (autism and ID). These observations led to the delineation of diagnostic criteria for individuals with a wide range of impairments beginning in DSM-III-R (APA, 1987) and the inclusion of a mild variant, Asperger's Disorder, as a separate diagnosis beginning in DSM-IV (APA, 1994). Current criteria for Asperger's Disorder (AsD) emphasize impairments in social interaction and nonverbal communication similar to autism but without delays in cognition or language development (Klin, Volkmar, Sparrow, Cicchetti, & Rourke, 1995). Because of the large overlap with autism, much ongoing investigation centers on whether Asperger's Disorder should be a separate classification or should be considered simply a mild form of autism.

ASSOCIATED FEATURES AND COMORBID CONDITIONS

Researchers have identified many other characteristics that are common but not universal (DSM-IV-TR, 2000). Most display a scatter in abilities (e.g., visual motor skills more advanced than language and social skills). Approximately 10 percent show splinter skills (i.e., skills that are far more advanced than their overall developmental level) such as precocious reading, rapid mathematical calculations, or strong memory for particular facts. Most, however, show significant and pervasive cognitive delays with approximately 75 percent of individuals with autism also diagnosed with ID (APA, 2000).

Behavioral difficulties are frequent, with more than 90 percent having tantrums of some form and perhaps 10 to 20 percent engaging in either self-injurious or aggressive behaviors (e.g., Lovaas, 1987). Many children with autism also display overactivity, unusually picky eating habits, problems initiating and maintaining sleep, difficulty with transitions, negative reactions to even slight changes in the environment, and atypical sensory responses such as apparent unresponsiveness to sounds or pain stimuli (APA, 2000).

Compared to typically developing children, children with autism may be at greater risk for attention deficit hyperactivity disorder (ADHD), affective disorders, anxiety disorders, and Tourette disorder (Tsai, 1996). Cross-sectional studies show age-related differences in the clinical symptoms over time with attention problems giving way to anxiety and depressive symptoms (Tsai, 1996). Since studies on comorbid conditions have been rare, precise estimates of their prevalence among individuals with autism are unavailable.

ETIOLOGY

Autism appears to be a neurobiological disorder with a strong genetic basis. The disorder clusters in families, and the risk for a particular family member is linked to the genetic similarity of the affected individual. Identical twins share 100% of their genes; when one identical twin has autism, the risk for the other is approximately 60% (rising as high as 93% if milder variants such as Asperger's Disorder are included; Bailey et al., 1995). Siblings share 50% of their genes; when one sibling has autism, the risk for the other is about 3 to 7% (Simonoff, 1998). Recently, investigators have identified several genes that may confer vulnerability to autism, although replications are needed (Nicolson & Szatmari, 2003).

Despite varied results, most brain imaging studies suggest that individuals with autism have an enlarged brain (Bauman & Kemper, 1995) but decreased volume and activity in specific areas: (a) the cerebellum (Courschesne, Yeung-Courschesne, Press, Hesselink, & Jernigan, 1988), which may be involved in sequencing activities such as a series of motor movements (e.g., grooming and hygiene activities, sports etc.), (b) posterior hippocampus (Saitoh, Courschesne, Egaas, Lincoln, & Schiebman, 1995), which may be associated with complex (non-rote) learning, (c) the amygdala (Baron-Cohen, Ring, Bullmore, Wheelwright, Ashwin, & Williams, 2000), which may contribute to recognizing faces and decoding emotional expressions, and (d) several structures in the brain stem (Rodier, 2000) that are associated with attention. Research also indicates that individuals with autism have high levels of the neurotransmitter serotonin (Hashino et al., 1994) that may be associated with behaviors such as stereotypy (e.g., repetitive behaviors such as hand-flapping, body-rocking etc.). However, given that findings on brain structure and activity have not been consistently replicated, the etiology of autism remains incompletely understood.

A few investigators believe the recent rise in prevalence estimates for autism reflects an actual increase in the disorder, and they implicate toxins in foods (Reichelt, Knivsberg, Lindberg, & Noland, 1991), vaccines (Wakefield et al., 1998), and pollutants (Agency for Toxic Substances and Disease Registry, 1999). However, most evidence indicates that autism is unrelated to these substances (Centers for Disease Control, 2000).

COURSE AND IMPACT

Autism begins prior to age 3 and is almost always a life-long condition. Most individuals with autism can improve with age and intervention. About 10% can be considered to have a "good" outcome; that is, they develop language and social skills and make adequate progress in school or work, but they may continue to show abnormalities in speech and social behavior. Another 20% are considered to have "fair" outcomes, and 70% have "poor" or "very poor" outcomes, with limited progress across many developmental areas leaving them severely handicapped (e.g., Gillberg & Steffenburg, 1987). These outcome statistics appear to correspond to the percent of individuals with autism that also have ID, suggesting that intellectual and language deficits can moderate the amount of progress that an individual with autism can make.

In adolescence, many individuals with autism display more interest in social interaction. Up to one-third show increased hyperactivity and compulsive or repetitive behaviors, and roughly one-quarter develop seizures that persist into adulthood (Gillberg & Steffenburg, 1987). As adults, some maintain jobs and a few (perhaps 5%) live independently, succeed in skilled occupations, and establish meaningful social relationships (APA, 1994).

Given that autism usually co-occurs with ID and is frequently also accompanied by other behavior disturbances, it has a substantial impact on the family. Families may incur both emotional and financial costs when caring for an individual with autism. Parents, especially mothers, experience elevated levels of parenting stress, burden, and marital strain relative to parents of children with other chronic illnesses (Fisman, Wolf, & Noh, 1989; Hoppes & Harris, 1990; Rodrigue, Morgan, & Gefkin, 1990), including Down syndrome (Holroyd & McArthur, 1976). These problems may also compromise the parents' own emotional well-being. Not all families can provide care for the entire life of a relative with autism. About half of the adults with autism live in residential care (Seltzer, Krauss, Orsmond, & Vestal 2001). Applied behavior analytic (ABA) treatment, when implemented intensively (more than 20 hours per week) and early (beginning prior to age 5), may substantially decrease the number of individuals with autism who require residential care as adults (Jacobson, Mulick, & Green, 1998).

TREATMENT OF AUTISM

Currently, autism is a treatable but incurable disorder. Applied behavior analysis (ABA) treatment is the primary empirically supported intervention (e.g., National Research Council, 2001; Green, 1996), although higher functioning individuals may also benefit from clinical behavior therapy (Tsai, 1999). Medications may be useful in some cases for management of core clinical difficulties (e.g., repetitive and stereotyped behaviors) and associated features (e.g., anxiety, depression, aggression, and self-injury) and when combined with behavioral intervention. In addition, many other interventions, individual therapies, and biological remedies have become widespread, despite an absence of controlled studies on their effectiveness.

Behavioral treatments significantly improve skills in such areas as receptive and expressive language (Goldstein, 2002), self-help, play activities (e.g., McClannahan & Krantz, 1999; Pierce & Schreibman, 1994) and social skills (McConnell, 2002). Many children with autism also acquire functional reading and mathematics, and most learn vocational skills such as assembly and filing tasks (e.g., Etzel, Leblanc, Schillmoeller, & Steller, 1981). In addition, behavioral intervention reduces disruptive or problematic behaviors (Matson, Benavidez, Compton, Paclawskyj, & Baglio, 1996).

ABA can be applied to teach specific skills or to provide comprehensive intervention. Specific skill models are most often appropriate for individuals who have autism without comorbid conditions; comprehensive models are designed for individuals with co-occurring autism and ID, as such individuals require intensive and broad skill development (discussed below in "Treatment for Co-occurring Autism and ID"). The main specific skill models are parent training, consultation to educational or residential settings, and clinical behavior therapy.

Parent training involves providing 20-50 hours of instruction in ABA approaches to enable families to teach skills in the home. Investigators such as Jocelyn, Casiro, Beattie, Bow, & Kneisz (1998) have reported that parents who receive this instruction successfully teach a variety of skills to their children. Koegel, Schreibman, Britten, Burke, & O'Neill (1982) found that parent training was more effective than five hours per week of direct instruction to the child with autism from ABA providers.

Consultation to educational or residential settings includes:
- Training educational personnel on autism and effective, evidenced-based educational approaches;
- Establishing teamwork among behavioral practitioners, school personnel, and families;
- Integrating ABA instructional approaches into the general educational curriculum, and
- Augmenting in-school supports for the individual with autism (e.g., teaching the available speech and language pathologist to conduct social skills training and setting up peer networks; problem-solving with the teacher; Klin & Volkmar, 2000).

School personnel learn to use direct instruction and incidental teaching to assist students with autism in particular areas such as peer interaction, self-management, self-instruction, self-control, and daily living skills. They also learn to adapt the academic curriculum and expand instructional strategies to create opportunities for a successful educational experience. For example, providing a daily schedule on the student's desk may facilitate transitions between activities, and giving instructions visually rather than orally may improve the student's performance (Janney & Snell, 2000). As students approach adulthood, the focus is increasingly on identifying jobs that fit their interests and abilities and providing instruction in areas such as interviewing skills, grooming and hygiene, and social skills (Klin & Volkmar, 2000). Many studies document that individuals with autism acquire skills when educational and residential personnel receive consultation on ABA (Matson et al., 1996). However, little research has been conducted examining long-term outcomes of these interventions, particularly for adolescents and adults.

Individuals with autism, who have extensive language skills, may benefit from cognitive and clinical behavior therapies that focus on social communication skills (Minskoff, 1987, 1994), stress management, problem-solving, and social perspective taking (i.e., Theory of Mind: Howlin, Baron-Cohen, & Hadwin, 1999; Ozonoff & Miller, 1995). These therapies can be conducted individually (e.g., Howlin, Baron-Cohen, & Hadwin, 1999) or in groups (e.g.,

Ozonoff & Miller, 1995). Studies indicate that the therapies promote acquisition of skills, but that the skills often do not generalize to everyday settings (Ozonoff & Miller, 1995).

TREATMENT OF CO-OCCURING AUTISM AND INTELLECTUAL DISABILITY

ABA is the intervention with the most extensive empirical support for individuals with co-occurring autism and ID. However, many other educational models, individual therapies, and biological remedies are in widespread use despite an absence of controlled studies on their effectiveness. Those interventions will be reviewed at the end of this section.

Several considerations are unique to ABA interventions with this population. First, research indicates that these individuals may benefit from early intervention (beginning prior to the age of 4 years) to a greater extent than do individuals with other developmental disabilities (Guralnick, 1998). As a result, early intensive behavioral intervention (EIBI) is a top priority. Second, many individuals with autism and ID enter treatment with extremely limited social and communication skills. Therefore, they require especially comprehensive instruction in these areas. Instruction often begins with basic skills such as imitating an individual action performed by a model or responding to a one-word request and proceeding in a systematic, stepwise manner to more complex skills (Newsom, 1998). Third, at the start of treatment, individuals with autism and ID are likely to be extremely inattentive, make active attempts to escape, or engage in ritualistic behaviors. For this reason, they are more likely to require highly structured teaching methods such as discrete trial training (DTT), than most other individuals with developmental disabilities (Smith, 2001). Finally, as previously noted, stress is often acute in families of individuals with autism. Consequently, ABA for individuals with autism places a particularly strong emphasis on involving parents in treatment.

EIBI for Young Children

This approach emphasizes two to three years of intensive behavioral intervention (20 or more hours per week) prior to age 5, followed by a continuation of behavioral treatment in the special or regular education classroom for those school-aged children that require additional intervention. Treatment progresses in stages and varies in length depending on the individual's skill level and response to treatment. The beginning stage has two interdependent goals: 1) teaching behaviors that promote learning (e.g., attending behavior) and 2) reducing behaviors that interfere with learning (e.g., non-compliance, withdrawal, self-injury). Discrete trial teaching (DTT) procedures teach learning readiness skills while reductive procedures (usually differential reinforcement and extinction) are used to treat interfering behaviors. This phase of treatment establishes the social context for the child and helps the child to distinguish adults as consistent sources of positive and negative consequences. It also introduces the child to the teaching framework (stimulus-response-consequence) that many subsequent teaching interactions will apply (Newsom, 1998).

The next phase of treatment seeks to expand the child's basic skills into more complex language, play, and social repertoires. Daily living skills are also targeted for development. During this phase, the child is taught to follow instruction, request preferred items/activities, ask questions, match objects and pictures, identify numbers and letters, play with toys functionally, interact with peers, draw and write, eat independently, and assist with basic grooming and hygiene. Various teaching procedures are used to train skills in these areas including discrete trial teaching, incidental teaching, direct instruction, shaping and chaining.

For many children, the final phase of their treatment will focus on the development of higher-level skills such as observational learning, problem-solving, coping, self-management, and classroom participation skills. This training seeks to prepare the child for placement into the public school setting. However, for other children, additional treatment is necessary upon entry into the public school. Here, treatment focuses on the further development of the child's social communication skills, academic skills, and classroom participation skills, with the goal of teaching the child in the least restrictive educational environment (Smith, Magyar, & Arnold-Saritepe, 2002).

A team of individuals that includes the parents, psychologist or behavior analyst, special education teacher, speech and language pathologist, and paraprofessional skill instructor usually delivers the EIBI treatment. While early phases of treatment generally take place in the child's home, eventual participation in a school-based program and the inclusion of peers into treatment is considered essential.

Research has demonstrated that EIBI enables many children with autism to make major developmental gains in IQ and language. It has also been shown to foster improvements in socio-emotional functioning and participation in inclusive school placements (see Smith, 1999 for a review). While there continues to be large individual differences in response to EIBI, as evidenced by some children who make very significant improvements, while others appear to benefit little; many believe that treatment may be appropriate for most children with autism who are under 5 years (New York State Department of Health, 1999).

ABA for Older Individuals

Individuals with co-occurring autism and ID, who respond favorably to ABA, may attain age-appropriate levels of functioning in many areas and require few ongoing services (McEachin, Smith, & Lovaas, 1993). Individuals who respond less favorably or who do not receive EIBI are likely to require ongoing intervention as they enter elementary school and continue to need such intervention as they grow older. The intervention may consist of placement in a public school setting with ABA consultation, as described in the preceding section (Smith, Magyar, & Arnold-Saritepe, 2002). Alternatively, it may involve placement in a self-contained ABA program. At present, this placement decision is based on clinical judgment, as there are not established evidence-based guidelines.

In ABA programs, instructors continue to work on expanding skills for communication, social interaction, play activities, and self-care. Also, there is increasing emphasis placed on individuals performing tasks without adult supervision. For example, to teach individuals to perform a variety of leisure, self-care, and occupational tasks, they are taught to follow schedules presented in pictures (McClannahan, MacDuff, & Krantz, 2002). In addition, they receive extensive vocational training with the goal of securing employment in the community (Holmes, 1997). As is true of specific skills programs, the effectiveness of comprehensive ABA programs for teaching skills to older individuals with autism is well documented (Matson et al., 1996), but, particularly for adolescents and adults, long-term outcomes need much additional research.

Alternatives or Supplements to ABA

In addition to ABA, two other educational interventions for children who have autism, with or without ID, have been developed and evaluated in peer-reviewed studies: Project TEACCH and the Denver Model. In Project TEACCH (Treatment and Education of Autistic and Communication-Handicapped Children; Schopler & Olley, 1980), individuals with autism receive classroom instruction that is designed to accommodate the learning disabilities associated with the disorder. The program incorporates some behavioral procedures like prompts and reinforcement, mainly for teaching self-care skills and managing problem behavior, but does not endorse the application of many other behavioral methods to teach other skills like language, academics, social skills, or play skills.

The primary teaching strategy, called structured teaching, is essentially a system for organizing the classroom so that the student can make clear associations between specific areas of the room and corresponding activities. To assist the student to follow the classroom routine and predict upcoming events, visual schedules depicting the sequence of events in a given day, period of the day, or week are developed and displayed in prominent locations. Schedules are designed not only for assisting the student in following a routine but also for reducing anxiety associated with making transitions from one activity to another. Individual work systems are designed to provide the student with information about the type and amount of work that needs to be completed and what will occur when the work is finished (Mesibov, Schopler, & Hearsey, 1994). Visual organizational strategies are used to focus attention on important aspects of the environment by making salient certain vital features of the teaching materials and aspects of the work task. A number of uncontrolled and quasi-experimental studies suggest that Project TEACCH is effective. However, no controlled studies currently exist (Smith, 1999).

In the Denver Model (Rogers, Hall, Osaki, Reaven, & Herbison, 2000), the aim is to establish a nurturing, reciprocal relationship with the individual with autism. By encouraging the individual to choose activities, ask to finish activities, and take turns in games and songs, the teacher seeks to teach communication, independent living, social, and classroom participation skills. Uncontrolled studies indicate that individuals with autism may demonstrate gains on developmental testing after participating in the Denver Model, but this finding has not yet been confirmed in controlled investigations (Smith, 1999).

Another influential model is Greenspan's Developmental Individual-Difference Relationship-Based Model (DIR; Greenspan & Weider, 1999). The goal of treatment is to re-establish the individual's ability to engage in interpersonal communication. There are three main therapeutic components: Floor Time, semi-structured problem-solving, and semi-structured sensory activities. In Floor Time, caregivers follow their child's lead and aim to establish a back-and-forth flow of communication by using interventions such as playfully obstructing a child's behavior (e.g., a caregiver uses her arms to build a fence around a child who likes to run away). Problem-solving includes activities designed to foster reasoning and language development. Semi-structured activities may include sensory integration therapy, perceptual-motor challenges such as looking/doing games, visual-spatial activities such as obstacle courses, and tactile discrimination such as finding objects hidden in materials with different textures.

Although DIR has not been evaluated in controlled research to date, many of the strategies used in DIR parallel certain behavioral techniques that have been shown to be effective (e.g., incidental teaching, prompt and fade techniques, differential reinforcement for other behavior), and therefore DIR deserves empirical investigation.

Sensory motor therapies are a popular supplement to educational programs. Proponents contend that individuals with autism have deficits in sensory perception that hinder them from modulating the intensity or variety of sensory stimuli from their environment. In this view, individuals with autism resort to behaviors like self-injury or ritualistic behavior in an attempt to compensate for their atypical processing of sensory stimuli. Sensory Integration Therapy (SIT; Ayres, 1972, 1974) has been especially influential. The aim of SIT is to improve sensory processing in the brain by stimulating the vestibular system and skin. For example, deep-joint compression, body-squeezing, and jumping are activities for enhancing the vestibular system. Running a soft-bristled brush back and forth along the arms, legs, and back provides tactile input to an individual's skin. Although many people with autism and other developmental disabilities have received SIT since the early 1970s, evidence of the effectiveness of SIT consists mainly of subjective reports. The few well-controlled studies indicate that SIT is ineffective (Smith, Mruzek, & Mozingo, 2003).

TREATMENT FOR AUTISM AND OTHER CO-OCCURRING CONDITIONS

In addition to educational intervention, ABA is often effective in reducing maladaptive behaviors associated with autism such as tantrums, aggression, self-injury, running away, deregulated sleep, or picky eating (Matson et al., 1996). Prior to intervention, a functional behavior analysis is conducted to identify environmental events that appear to trigger or reinforce the behavior. From this analysis, an intervention is derived that includes procedures for both reducing the maladaptive behavior (e.g., extinction) and for teaching adaptive skills that may replace the behavior (see Chapter 8 of this volume). ABA can also been used to decrease anxiety; relaxation training can be effective for individuals with autism (e.g., Love, Matson, & West, 1990).

Some medications ameliorate mental disorders or behavioral disturbances associated with autism, though they have little impact on the core disturbances in communication and socialization. The best-studied medication is the atypical neuroleptic, risperidone. A large, well-designed clinical trial revealed that this medication alleviated severe behavior disturbances (e.g., aggression, non-compliance) in more than two-thirds of children with autism who displayed them (McCracken et al., 2002). In some cases, selective serotonin reuptake inhibitors such as fluoxetine and sertraline reduce repetitive and compulsive behaviors, aggression, and social isolation (McDougle et al., 1992; Aman, Arnold, & Armstrong, 1999). Medications that influence epinephrine or norepinephrine such as clonidine may curtail self-injurious behavior and/or aggression and hyperarousal (Jaselskis, Cook, Fletcher, & Leventhal, 1992). Also, naltrexone has been reported to have some therapeutic effect in reducing aggression, self-injury, and hyperactivity and in increasing social behaviors (Campbell et al., 1993). Finally, methylphenidate may reduce ADHD behaviors, particularly in individuals without ID (Aman, 1996). However, medications may be more effective for adults with autism rather than children, (Tsai, 1999), and few studies have assessed long-term outcomes.

Additional biological interventions such as megavitamins have been used to treat behavioral disturbances such as hyperactivity and sensory-motor abnormalities. Over a dozen published studies have reported improvements in individuals treated with high-dose

Vitamin B6 and magnesium. However, these studies have had significant methodological difficulties, and well-designed studies have indicated that B6 with magnesium may not be effective (for a review, see Singh, Ellis, Mulick, & Poling, 1998). Other supplements have been used to treat sleep difficulties and include the hormone melatonin (Jan & O'Donnell, 1996) and the oral antihistamine, niaprazine (Rossi, Posar, Parmeggiani, Pipitone & Agata, 1999).

SUMMARY

Many advances have occurred in elucidating the behavioral characteristics of autism, the prevalence of the disorder, co-occurring conditions, course and impact on affected individuals and family members, possible etiologic mechanisms, and effective interventions. However, a number of issues remain unresolved. It is unclear whether autism and autistic spectrum disorders such as Asperger's Disorder are distinct conditions or merely different manifestations of the same condition. Also, it is uncertain why the reported prevalence of autism has increased in recent years. Broader diagnostic criteria have certainly contributed to this increase, but investigators are also studying whether other factors are involved. A paucity of information exists on the rate of co-occurring conditions other than ID. In addition, although several candidate genes and neurological mechanisms have been identified, the precise etiology or etiologies of autism continue to elude investigators. The large individual differences in response to treatments such as ABA are another enigma. Moreover, investigators have tended to focus on evaluating interventions for children with autism rather than adolescents or adults. For this reason, best practices for older individuals with autism are not well specified. Further, most treatment studies have focused on child outcomes rather than family outcomes. Thus, the impact of treatment on the family is undetermined. Long-term outcome of treatment for co-occurring conditions (e.g., ADHD) is another topic that is essentially unexplored. The resolution of these issues is a top priority for future research.

REFERENCES

Agency for Toxic Substances and Disease Registry. (1999). Public Health Assessment: Brick Township Assessment. Access: http:/www.atsdr.cdc.gov/HAC/PHA/bri/bri_toc.html

Aman, M. G. (1996). Stimulant drugs in the developmental disabilities revisited. *Journal of Developmental and Physical Disabilities, 8*, 347-365.

Aman, M. G., Arnold, L. E., & Armstrong, S. C. (1999). Review of serotonergic agents and perseverative behavior in patients with developmental disabilities. *Mental Retardation and Developmental Disabilities Research Reviews, 5*, 279-289.

American Psychiatric Association. (1980). *Diagnostic and statistical manual of mental disorders* (3rd ed.). Washington, DC.

American Psychiatric Association. (1987). *Diagnostic and statistical manual of mental disorders* (Rev. 3rd ed.). Washington, DC.

American Psychiatric Association. (1994). *Diagnostic and statistical manual of mental disorders* (4th ed.). Washington, DC.

American Psychiatric Association. (2000). *Diagnostic and statistical manual of mental disorders* (Rev. 4th ed.). Washington, DC.

Ayres, A. J. (1972). *Sensory integration and learning disorders*. Los Angeles: Western Psychological Services.

Ayres, A. J. (1974). *The development of sensory integrative theory and practice*. Dubuque, IA: Kendall/Hunt.

Bailey, A., LeCouteru, A., Gottesman, I., Bolton, P., Simonoff, E., Yuzda, E., et al. (1995). Autism is a strongly genetic disorder: Evidence from a British twin study. *Psychological Medicine, 25*, 63-77.

Baron-Cohen, S., Ring, H. A., Bullmore, E. T., Wheelwright, S., Ashwin, C., & Williams, S. C. (2000). The amygdala theory of autism. *Neuroscience and Biobehavioral Reviews, 24*, 355-364.

Bauman, M. L., & Kemper, T. L. (1994). Neuroanatomic observations of the brain in autism. In M. L. Bauman & T. L. Kemper (Eds.), *The neurobiology of autism* (pp. 119-145). Baltimore: Johns Hopkins University Press.

Bettelheim, B. (1967). *The empty fortress*. New York: Free Press.

Bleuler, E. (1950). *Dementia praecox* (J. Zinkin, Trans.). New York: International Universities Press. (Original work published 1911)

Bouma, R., & Schweitzer, R. (1990). The impact of chronic childhood illness on family stress: A comparison between autism and cystic fibrosis. *Journal of Clinical Psychology, 46*, 722-730.

Bryson, S., & Smith, I. (1998). Epidemiology of autism: Prevalence, associated characteristics, and implications for research and service delivery. *Mental Retardation and Developmental Disabilities Research Reviews, 4*, 97-103.

Campbell, M., Anderson, L. T., Small, A. M., Adams, P., Gonzalez, N. M., & Ernst, M. (1993). Naltrexone in autistic children: Behavioral symptoms and attentional learning. *Journal of American Academy of Child and Adolescent Psychiatry, 32*, 1283-1291.

Courschesne, E., Yeung-Courschesne, R., Press, G. A., Hesselink, J. R., & Jernigan, T. L. (1988). Hypoplasia of cerebellar vermal lobules VI and VII in autism. *New England Journal of Medicine, 318*, 1349-1354.

DeMyer, M., Pontius, W., Norton, J., Barton, S., & Steele, R. (1972). Parental practices and innate activity in autistic and brain-damaged infants. *Journal of Autism and Childhood Schizophrenia, 2*, 49-66.

Education for All Handicapped Children Act (EAHCA), 20 U.S.C, Secs. 1400 et seq. (1975).

Etzel, B. C., Leblanc, J. M., Schillmoeller, K. J., & Stella, M. E. (1981). Behavior Modification contributions to education. In Bijou, S. W. & Ruiz, R. (Eds.), *Stimulus control procedures in the education of young children* (pp 3-37). Hillsdale, NJ: Lawrence Erlbaum.

Fisman, S. N., Wolf, L. C., & Noh, S. (1989). Marital intimacy in parents of exceptional children. *Canadian Journal of Psychiatry, 34*, 519-525.

Gillberg, C., & Steffenburg, S. (1987). Outcome and prognostic factors in infantile autism and similar conditions: A population-based study of 46 cases followed through puberty. *Journal of Autism and Developmental Disorders, 17*, 273-287.

Goldstein, H. (2002). Communication intervention for children with autism: A review of treatment efficacy. *Journal of Autism and Developmental Disorders, 32*, 373-396.

Greenspan, S. I., & Wieder, S. (1999). A functional developmental approach to autism spectrum disorders. *Journal of the Association for Persons with Severe Handicaps, 24*, 147-161.

Guralnick, M. J. (1998). Effectiveness of early intervention for vulnerable children: A developmental perspective. *American Journal on Mental Retardation, 102*, 319-345.

Holmes, D. (1997). *Autism through the lifespan: The Eden Model.* Bethesda, MD: Woodbine House.

Holroyd, J., & McArthur, D. (1976). Mental retardation and stress on the parents: A contrast between Down syndrome and childhood autism. *American Journal of Mental Deficiency, 80*, 431-436.

Hoppes, K., & Harris, S. L. (1990). Perceptions of child attachment and maternal gratification in mothers of children with autism and Down's syndrome. *Journal of Clinical Child Psychology, 19*, 365-370.

Hoshino, Y., Yamamoto, T., Kaneko, M., Tachibana, R., Watanabe, M., Ono., Y., et al. (1984). Blood serotonin and free tryptophan concentration in autistic children. *Neuropsychobiology, 11*, 22-27.

Howlin, P. A., & Rutter, M. (1987). *Treatment of autistic children.* New York: Wiley.

Jacobson, J. W., Mulick, J. A., & Green, G. (1998). Cost-benefit estimates for early intensive behavioral intervention for young children with autism: General models and single state case. *Behavioral Interventions, 13*, 201-226.

Jan, J. E., & O'Donnell, M.E. (1996). Use of melatonin in the treatment of pediatric sleep disorders. *Journal of Pineal Research, 21*, 193-199.

Janney, R., & Snell, N. E. (2000). *Teacher's guide to inclusive practices: Modifying schoolwork.* Baltimore: Paul H. Brookes.

Jaselskis, C. A., Cook, E. H., Fletcher, K. E., & Leventhal, B. L. (1992). Clonidine treatment of hyperactive and impulsive children with autistic disorder. *Journal of Clinical Psychopharmacology, 12*, 322-327.

Jocelyn, L. J., Casiro, O. G, Beattie, D., Bow, J., & Kneisz, J. (1998). Treatment of children with autism: A randomized controlled trial to evaluate a caregiver-based intervention program in community day-care centers. *Journal of Developmental & Behavioral Pediatrics, 19*, 326-334.

Kanner, L. (1943). Autistic disturbances of affective contact. *Nervous Child, 2,* 217-250.

Klin, A., & Volkmar, F. R. (2000). Treatment and intervention guidelines for individuals with Asperger Syndrome. In A. Klin, F. R. Volkmar, & S. S. Sparrow (Eds.), *Asperger Syndrome* (pp. 340-366). New York: Guilford.

Klin, A., Volkmar, F. R., Sparrow, S. S., Cicchetti, D. V., & Rourke, B. P. (1995). Validity and neuropsychological characterization of Asperger syndrome: Convergence with nonverbal learning disabilities syndrome. Journal of Child Psychology and Psychiatry, *36*, 1127-1140.

Koegel, R. L., Schreibman, L., Britten, K. R., Burke, J. C., & O'Neill, R. E. (1982). A comparison of parent training to direct child treatment. In R. L. Koegel, A. Rincover, & A. L. Egel (Eds.), *Educating and understanding autistic children* (pp. 260-279). San Diego, CA: College Hill Press.

Kolvin, I., Ounsted, C., Humphrey, M., McNay, A., Richardson, L. M., Garside, R. F., et al. (1971). Six studies in childhood psychoses. *British Journal of Psychiatry, 118*, 381-419.

Lovaas, O. I., Berberich, J. P., Perloff, B. F., & Schaeffer, B. (1966). Acquisition of imitative speech by schizophrenic children. *Science, 151*, 705-707.

Love, S. R., Matson, J. L., West, D. (1990). Mothers as effective therapists for autistic children's phobias. *Journal of Applied Behavior Analysis, 23*, 379-385.

Matson, J., Benavidez, D., Compton, L., Paclawskyj, T., & Baglio, C. (1996). Behavioral treatment of autistic persons: A review of research from 1980 to the present. *Research in Developmental Disabilities, 17*, 433-465.

McClannahan, L. E., & Krantz, P. J. (1999). *Activity schedules for children with autism: Teaching independent behavior.* New Jersey: Woodbine House.

McClannahan, L. E., MacDuff, G. S., & Krantz, P. J. (2002). Behavior analysis and intervention for adults with autism. *Behavior Modification, 26*, 9-26.

McConnell, S. R. (2002). Interventions to facilitate social interaction for young children with autism: Review of available research and recommendations for educational intervention and future research. *Journal of Autism and Developmental Disorders, 32*, 351-372.

McCracken, J. T., McGough, J., Shah, B., Cronin, P., Hong, D., Aman, M. G., et al. (2002). Risperidone in children with autism and serious behavior problems. *The New England Journal of Medicine, 347*, 314-321.

McDougle, C. J. (1997). Psychopharmacology. In D. J. Cohen & F. R. Volkmar (Eds.), *Handbook of autism and pervasive developmental disorders* (2nd ed., 707-729). New York: John Wiley & Sons.

McEachin, J. J., Smith, T., & Lovaas, O. I. (1993). Long-term outcome for children with autism who received early intensive behavioral treatment. *American Journal on Mental Retardation, 97*, 359-372.

Mesibov, G. B., Schopler, E., & Hearsey, K. A. (1994). Structured teaching. In E. Schopler & G. B. Mesibov (Eds.), *Behavioral issues in autism.* New York: Plenum.

National Research Council (2001). *Educating children with autism.* Committee on Educational Interventions for Children with Autism. Division of Behavioral and Social Sciences and Education. Washington, DC: National Academy Press.

New York State Department of Health (1999). Clinical practice guideline, Report of Recommendations – Early Intervention Program: Autism and Pervasive Developmental Disorders. Access http://www.health.state.ny.us/nysdoh/eip/autism/index.html

Newsom, C. B. (1998). Autistic disorder. In E. J. Mash & R. A. Barkley, (Eds.), *Treatment of childhood disorders,* (2nd ed., pp. 416-467). New York: Guilford Press.

Nicolson, R., & Szatmari, P. (2003). Genetic and neurodevelopmental influences in autistic disorder. *Canadian Journal of Psychiatry, 8*, 526-537.

Ozonoff, S., & Miller, J. N. (1995). Teaching theory of mind: A new approach to social skills training for individuals with autism. *Journal of Autism and Developmental Disorders, 25*, 415-433.

Pierce, K. L., & Schreibman, L. (1994). Teaching daily living skills to children with autism in unsupervised settings through pictorial self-management. *Journal of Applied Behavior Analysis, 27,* 471-481.

Reichelt, K. L., Knivsberg, A. M., Lind, G., & Nodland, M. (1991). Probable etiology and possible treatment of childhood autism. *Brain Dysfunction, 4*, 308-319.

Rodier, P. M. (2000). The early origins of autism. *Scientific American, 282(2),* 56-63.

Rodrigue, J. R., Morgan, S. B., & Geffken, G. (1990). Families of autistic children: Psychological functioning of mothers. *Journal of Clinical Child Psychology, 19*, 371-379.

Rogers, S. J., Hall, T., Osaki, D., Reaven, J., & Herbison, J. (2000). The Denver Model: A comprehensive, integrated educational approach to young children with autism. In J. S. Handleman & S. L. Harris (Eds.), *Preschool programs for children with autism* (2nd ed., pp. 95-134). Austin, TX: Pro-Ed.

Rossi, P. G., Posar, A., Parmeggiani, A., Pipitone, D. S., & D'Agata, M. (1999). Niaprazine in the treatment of autistic disorder. *Journal of Child Neurology, 14*, 547-550.

Rutter, M., Bartak, L., & Newman, S. (1971). Autism: Central disorder of cognition and language? In M. Rutter (Ed.), *Infantile autism: Concepts, characteristics, and treatment* (pp. 148-151). London: Churchill-Livingstone.

Rutter, M. (1972). Childhood Schizophrenia reconsidered. *Journal of Autism and Childhood Schizophrenia, 2*, 315-337.

Saitoh, O., Courschesne, E., Egaas, B., Lincoln, A. J., & Schiebman, L. (1995). Cross-sectional area of the posterior hippocampus in autistic patients with cerebellar and corpus callosum abnormalities. *Neurology, 45*, 317-345.

Schopler, E., & Mesibov, G. B. (Eds.). (1983). *Autism in adolescents and adults.* New York: Plenum Press.

Schopler, E. & Olley, J. G. (1980). Public school programming for autistic children. *Exceptional Children, 46,* 461-463.

Seltzer, M. M., Krauss, M. W., Orsmond, G. I., & Vestal, C. (2001). Families of adolescents and adults with autism: Uncharted territory. In L. M. Glidden (Ed.), *International Review of Research in Mental Retardation (Vol. 23): Autism* (pp. 267-294). San Diego, CA: Academic Press.

Simonoff, E. (1998). Genetic counseling in autism and pervasive developmental disorders. *Journal of Autism and Developmental Disorders, 28,* 447-456.

Singh, N. N., Ellis, C. R., Mulick, J. A., & Poling, A. (1998). Vitamin, mineral, and dietary treatments. In S. Reiss & M. G. Aman (Eds.), *Psychotropic medications and developmental disabilities.* Colombus, OH: The Ohio State University.

Smith, T. (1999). Outcome of early intervention for children with autism. *Clinical Psychology: Research and Practice, 6,* 33-49.

Smith, T. (2001). Discrete trial training in the treatment of autism. *Focus on Autism and Related Disorders, 16,* 86-92.

Smith, T., Magyar, C., & Arnold-Saritepe, A. (2002). Autism spectrum disorders. In D. Marsh & M. Fristad (Eds.), *Handbook of serious emotional disturbances of childhood* (pp. 131-148). New York: Wiley & Sons.

Smith, T., Mruzek, D., & Mozingo, D. (2003) (in press). Sensory Integrative Therapy. In J. W. Jacobson & R. M. Foxx (Eds.), *Fads, dubious and improbable treatments for developmental disabilities.* Mahwah, NJ: Laurence Erlbaum Associates.

Strain, P. S., & Kohler, F. (1999). Peer-mediated intervention for young children with autism: A 20-year retrospective. In P. M. Ghezzi, W. L. Williams, & J. E. Carr (Eds.), *Behavior analytic perspectives* (pp. 189-211). Reno, NV: Context Press.

Tsai, L.Y. (1999). Psychopharmacology in autism. *Psychosomatic Medicine, 61*, 651-681.

Tsai, L.Y. (1996). Comorbid psychiatric disorder of autistic disorders. *Journal of Autism and Developmental Disabilities, 26*, 159-163.

Wakefield, A. J., Murch, S. H., Anthony, A., Linnell, J., Casson, D. M., Malik, M., et al. (1998). Ileal-lymphoid-nodular hyperplasia, non-specific colitis, and pervasive developmental disorder in children. *Lancet, 351*, 637-641.

Author's Note

Caroline I. Magyar and Tristram Smith, Strong Center for Developmental Disabilities, Department of Pediatrics, University of Rochester Medical Center; Jennifer Katz, Department of Psychology, Rochester Institute of Technology

Address correspondence to Caroline I. Magyar, Ph.D. Strong Center for Developmental Disabilities, Department of Pediatrics, University of Rochester Medical Center, 601 Elmwood Avenue, Box 671, Rochester, NY 14642. Email: caroline_magyar@URMC.Rochester.edu.

7

Psychotherapeutic Interventions

JoAnne T. Baxter and Nancy N. Cain

INTRODUCTION

The concept of "normalization" is a term that originated in Sweden in the 1960s. Bengte Nirje (1969) defined normalization as "making available to the mentally retarded patterns and conditions of everyday life, which are as close as possible to the norms and patterns of mainstream society." Henry Cobb (1973) elaborated further on this concept by stating, "Essential to the normalization of the person is the reduction of all treatable conditions which impede normal functioning and the enhancement and functional utilization of all inherent capacities and potentialities of the person." Cobb's eloquent elaboration of normalization is applicable today in defining the ultimate goal that all service providers who work with individuals with ID should be striving toward. A mental disorder can prevent a person from attaining his or her goals and from fully enjoying life. Psychotherapy often plays an important role in ameliorating this. It can assist individuals with ID to identify their disability, come to accept it, distinguish what is unattainable, and identify what can be achieved to make the disability as non-handicapping as possible. It can help remove barriers between individuals with ID and the things that they want to do or attain.

The best, most comprehensive treatment for mental disorders is multifaceted. Psychotherapy is only one component of an integrated treatment plan that addresses all of the biopsychosocial interventions needed. It can augment or reinforce other components of therapy such as helping someone accept the need for medication. It can also be enhanced by other therapies. Behavior therapy may provide some structure needed to enable the individual to participate in the process of psychotherapy. A day treatment program can incorporate some of the psychotherapy goals and thus reinforce interpersonal growth and positive behavior changes and lead to greater success.

Until the 1980s it was believed that individuals with ID were unable to benefit from psychotherapy. If an individual presented with behavioral or emotional symptoms, the use of medication was the most frequently used intervention, especially if the individual was aggressive or disruptive.

Today, psychotherapy is viewed as a viable treatment for individuals with ID. They have responded positively to a variety of modalities, many of which will be discussed in this chapter.

Psychotherapy has assisted clients with ID to achieve significant improvement in their day-to-day functioning, leading to an overall improvement in their quality of life. Some of the benefits of therapy include:
- Improved self esteem;
- Improved interpersonal relationships;
- Increased use of effective coping skills;
- Increased ability to understand themselves and express their ideas more clearly;
- Heightened ability to express feelings or strong emotions verbally;
- Increased problem-solving skills;
- Development of more sophisticated decision-making skills;
- Increased ability to resolve conflict;
- Increased sense of empowerment;
- Greater ability to affect change, and
- Increased level of independence.

THE PROCESS OF PSYCHOTHERAPY

Often an eclectic approach, using a mixture of interventions, is most helpful. This gives the therapist the flexibility needed to increase the individual's ability to participate in and learn from the work. Modifying the approach to fit each client's level of understanding and ability to engage makes a positive outcome more likely. It is important to develop a therapeutic alliance or connection with the client. If this does not happen the client will not be an active participant, and any apparent changes will not be self-sustaining.

Not only do the various treatment modalities require modification, but the process of psychotherapy may also need some adaptations as well. Many aspects of psychotherapy with adults with ID are very similar to psychotherapy with children. Some examples of modification that may be needed include:
- Communication and collaboration with caregivers from all settings, including residential staff, day program staff, family members;
- Identify and prioritize goals through collaboration and consensus between the individual and caregivers;
- Educate the individual and caregivers about crucial aspects of therapy such as:
  - Confidentiality,
  - Patient rights,
  - Treatment planning process, and
  - Differences between therapy and other services.
- Therapist must communicate at individual's cognitive level;
- Therapist needs to be flexible, creative, and receptive to using a variety of treatment modalities, including individual therapy, group therapy, family therapy, and systems' approaches to ensure effective outcome.

Ellen Keller (2000) gives a comprehensive overview of these issues, including establishing a therapeutic alliance, educating individuals with ID about the therapeutic process, the development of goals, collaborating with systems, and the termination process.

It is important for therapists to have an awareness of common life experiences of individuals with ID in order to develop the genuine sense of empathy that is so crucial to the therapeutic relationship. Sovner & Hurley (1983); Judge (1983); Levitas & Gilson (1987), and Levitas & Gilson (1994) have provided insight into the obstacles and crises that individuals frequently encounter during their lifetime. Life transitions that are often unrecognized but can contribute to and increase emotional distress in adults with ID include:

- Graduation from school programs;
- Starting new work programs;
- Moving to new residential programs;
- Frequent staff turnover;
- Illness or death of parents, and
- Siblings surpassing them in developmental stages (e.g., dating, driving, going to college, getting married, having children).

TREATMENT MODALITIES

Transactional Analysis

"The goal of Transactional Analysis is to enable a person to have freedom of choice, freedom to change at will, and the ability to change the responses to recurring and new stimuli." (Harris, 1973). Eric Berne developed Transactional Analysis (TA). He defines a transaction as a stimulus from one person that produces a corresponding response in another (Kaplan & Sadock, 1991). Three ego states are described as making up the personality: the parent, the adult, and the child. The therapy involves helping the client understand the state in which he or she is in, when interacting with others. The goal is to have the client function as much as possible in the adult-ego state.

Phyllis Laterza (1983) cites the flexibility and easy comprehension of TA as the rationale for its use in the treatment of individuals with ID. The Parent-Adult-Child ego states are easily described, taught, and understood by clients. Although it may take more time to identify them with individuals with ID, this can be facilitated by the use of techniques from behavioral treatment such as role-playing and mirroring (see below). However, individuals with ID can learn to identify the ego state in which they are functioning, when exhibiting a particular behavior. This awareness can provide insight into particular transactions that they have with others, recognition of those relationships that cause conflict in their lives, and the ability to make decisions to change these patterns. Using TA techniques helps the individual look at his or her behavior, identify the appropriate ego state, and make decisions to think and behave in the adult mode. More Adult-to-Adult transactions lead to fewer behavior disturbances, have a positive effect on self-esteem, and can lead to a greater level of independence.

Example: Transactional Analysis

H. is a 35-year-old woman with mild ID and bipolar disorder. She has had a history of aggression, property destruction, "non-compliance," and running away. She came to her first appointment dressed in child-like attire including overall shorts, ruffled anklet socks, and a Winnie the Pooh baseball hat. As the session began, H. started to raise her voice and swear. She reported that she had been treated unfairly by staff, which prevented her from doing things the way that she wanted to, and had been supervised unnecessarily.

As therapy progressed she identified that she wished to increase her level of independence and improve her relationships with peers, staff, and family members. Therapy sessions then focused on educating and increasing H.'s understanding of the characteristics of the Parent-Adult-Child ego states. She began to discuss her outbursts that included behaviors such as whining, tantrums, and hitting others. In subsequent sessions, H. began to demonstrate the ability to consistently report these behaviors, understand how they impacted her interactions with others, and associate the various ego states with these interactions. H. began to develop an understanding that her pattern of child-like behavior, those of her "child ego state," often led to undesirable consequences such as being sent to her room or having increased supervision.

Regular review of H.'s interactions in various environments, both positive and negative, continued to increase her insight and awareness. Role-playing was an effective tool to practice alternative forms of expressing feelings, issues, and concerns in a manner that would illicit positive and desirable responses. She began talking about her concerns, stopped swearing and having tantrums, which had contributed to conflicts with other housemates, and was generally more aware of others. This led to improved relationships with peers, staff, family members; an improved self-image; a change in her choice in clothing, which became more age appropriate, and opportunities to increase her independence.

Laterza (1983) found that the concepts of TA could be simplified and explained to individuals with ID in concrete and easily understood terminology to enhance effectiveness. She reported that although the therapist needs to have "a more complex knowledge base of psychoanalytic and TA theory ... abstract conceptualization is not mandatory for the client to make gains in his or her developmental growth."

Modifications to traditional use of TA for individuals with ID include:
- Educate individual regarding the three ego states with simplified and concrete language geared to their cognitive level;
- Clear, concise examples of individual's behavior exemplifying the three ego states need to be repeated in an ongoing basis;
- Use of role-playing to practice changing behaviors and interactions with others, and
- Collaboration with care providers to assist with practicing role-plays outside the therapy sessions to facilitate generalization of new skills in all environmental settings.

Behavior Therapy

"The basic assumption of behavior therapy is that change of maladaptive behaviors can occur without insight into underlying causes" (Kaplan & Sadock, 1991). Specific behaviors are identified and programs developed to eliminate them. This therapy is based on operant and classical conditioning. Commonly used techniques with individuals with ID include: relaxation therapy, positive reinforcement, token economies, participant modeling, assertiveness training, and social skills training. (See Chapter 8 for a more in-depth discussion.)

Behavior contracts utilizing positive reinforcement have been helpful in promoting the frequency of more positive, prosocial behaviors while assisting in extinguishing inappropriate or less functional behaviors.

Hurley & Sovner (1986) define a reinforcer as "any event or thing, which occurs after a behavior is carried out and promotes an increase in the frequency of that behavior. It is the ability of the reinforcer to increase the rate at which the behavior occurs, not its rewarding value that is important in reinforcement procedures." They describe the following five steps to a successful implementation of a positive reinforcement behavioral plan:

- Include the individual in the treatment planning;
- Choose a target behavior to reinforce;
- Select an appropriate reinforcer;
- Ensure that the individual understands the behavior that is being reinforced, and
- Implement the program.

Programs need to be evaluated in terms of their effectiveness and changes made, if problems, or lack of effectiveness, are identified. Some common problems with plans are that reinforcers are not powerful enough, reinforcers are not consistently given, or there is confusion on the part of staff or the client on the implementation of the plan (Hurley et al., 1986). This type of therapy is frequently used in residential and day programs. It also can be quite effective as an adjunct to psychotherapy; an example of this follows:

Example 1: Behavior Therapy

K. is a 38-year-old woman who has moderate ID and a diagnosis of Mood Disorder NOS with psychotic features. She has a history of non-compliance and aggression. She has a boyfriend at her current group home and has difficulty separating from him to attend her group therapy sessions. These sessions have been important in keeping her stable and preventing regression. K. agreed to a contract in which she would attend her weekly group session and receive a certificate praising her for leaving her boyfriend, going to her group, and participating in therapy.

Relaxation

Relaxation is another component used in behavior therapy (see Chapter 8). Individuals with ID have demonstrated the ability to learn and to utilize some common relaxation techniques. The exercises need to be taught, demonstrated, and rehearsed frequently to be successfully internalized. Often clients will need verbal prompting, sometimes on an ongoing basis, to utilize these techniques at appropriate times. Some successfully used techniques include deep breathing exercises, counting to 10, and muscle relaxation with the use of a stress ball.

Role-playing

Role-playing is helpful to assist clients who have difficulty in the areas of assertiveness, social skills, and anger management. Individuals with ID often learn well through imitation and rehearsal. Mirroring is a technique that can be used to demonstrate to the individual some of their problematic behaviors. The therapist acts out exactly what the client does. This must not be done until there is a trusting relationship developed. It must be described clearly and over time before being implemented so that the client does not feel ridiculed. Modeling is another technique used in role-playing. Here, the therapist shows other, more appropriate or effective ways that the client may behave. All of this can then be practiced by having the client take one role and the therapist another so that the individual can learn the new behaviors. It must be practiced over and over to help the individual incorporate the behavior and to begin to recognize the different feeling that comes from it.

Example 2: Behavior Therapy

J. is a 30-year-old woman with mild ID. She has lived in a group home with 10 other people for the past eight years. One of her more disruptive behaviors was to yell and swear at staff when her demands where not met. At times, she would kick or hit them. Mirroring was used to help her begin to feel what it was like to have someone yell and swear at you in a menacing manner. She was able to recognize that this would not be the way to respond to authority figures such as her doctor. As she integrated this information, she could see that it was also inappropriate to do this with peers. She then began to role-play more appropriate ways to interact and communicate her feelings. After several sessions, she set a goal to recognize what her feelings were just before she became upset. At first she could only do this after the episode, but with support she began to learn what triggered the behaviors. Then she began using her new skills to respond more appropriately to staff. Developing a more positive relationship with the staff, ultimately reinforced her new skills. Once the "explosive" episodes stopped she became more eligible for a less restrictive residential setting and moved to a supervised apartment.

Cognitive Behavioral Therapy

"Cognitive therapy is based on the hypothesis that peoples' emotions and behaviors are influenced by their perceptions of events (Beck, 1995). Its overall goal is to identify and change distorted thoughts that maintain symptoms. It focuses on changing current behaviors by changing thoughts that are connected to these behaviors. This type of therapy is a frequently used intervention for Anger Management programs and the treatment of depression. Many behavioral techniques, such as the ones previously discussed, are used in connection with cognitive approaches.

Cognitive Behavioral Therapy (CBT) is a modality of treatment that:
- Usually is short term, 15 to 25 weeks;
- Focuses on present conflicts, feelings, issues;
- Emphasizes active participation of the individual;
- Teaches individuals how thoughts influence emotions, and

- Helps individuals identify, evaluate, and respond more appropriately to dysfunctional thoughts/beliefs (Beck 1995).

Some of the basic cognitive techniques that are utilized by the therapist to achieve identified goals include:
- Eliciting the individual's cognitive distortions, for example, " People will laugh at me when they see my new haircut";
- Identifying false assumptions by assisting the individual to identify patterns of thought, rules, and assumptions that cause such things as increased anxiety and depression, for example, "For people to like me I must never make a mistake," and
- Testing the validity of assumptions and cognitive distortions by having the individual explore reasons, for example, "Why can't you make a mistake?" (Kaplan & Sadock 1991).

Modifications are needed when using CBT with individuals with ID. In CBT individuals who do not have ID are required to "identify abstract concepts (*such as distorted ideas*), monitor and change their own behaviors, and identify patterns in their interactions" (Beck, 1995). Due to cognitive limitations and concrete thinking these aspects of treatment require changes to meet the developmental level of the client.

Modifications of CBT in treatment with individuals with ID include:
- Increasing the length of treatment to 1-2 years to achieve goals;
- Collaboration with staff and family members to assist individual and therapist in identifying distorted/irrational thoughts;
- Enlisting assistance from caregivers to assist the individual with completion of homework assignments, for example, rehearsing new responses via role-playing, and
- Building in positive reinforcements for completion of homework.

Example: Cognitive Behavior Therapy

H. is a 45-year-old man with mild ID who lives in a group home. He has a diagnosis of recurrent depression. When he is depressed he has difficulty and often refuses to get up in the morning. He often yells and swears at the staff when they try to get him out of bed. This leads to daily struggles between him and the staff.

H. comes from a family that was always criticizing and telling him what to do. His siblings are all married and doing well. He is often distressed when he thinks he is not living up to his family's expectations. His self-esteem is very fragile, and he experiences periods of increased negative self-image that manifests itself in the form of negative self-statements during his episodes of depression. After reviewing some of these thoughts with H. and connecting them with his behavior, he agreed to do daily homework to begin to change these thoughts. Each morning when he awoke he was to state three positive things about himself. Staff would prompt him to complete his homework and, if necessary, model some statements. Initially it was difficult for him to identify even one positive statement. With practice he became more successful. His self-esteem increased, his depression diminished, and he no longer had daily conflicts with the staff.

Psychodynamically Oriented Psychotherapy

"The aim of psychodynamically oriented therapy is to attempt to unblock developmental stalemates, to resolve unconscious emotional conflicts that constrict the individual options and life space, and to foster a capacity to love as well as work" (Ruth, 2001). It attempts to connect past, usually unconscious experiences with present behaviors and to change them. It is important to gain an understanding of the individual, his or her history, and of the interactions he or she has with the therapist.

Psychodynamically oriented therapy focuses on the impact that past experiences have on current problems. Its effectiveness is based on:
- Development of a non-judgmental, limit-setting environment;
- Use of clarification and interpretations;
- Enhancing an individual's ability to express feelings;
- Development of insight into the resemblance of the individual's responses to the therapist and responses in childhood situations;
- Increased awareness of distortions of previous experiences, relationships (Kaplan & Sadock 1991), and
- Insights into current interpersonal issues.

Though it was once believed that individuals with ID were not capable of benefiting from this type of therapy, due to their cognitive limitations, it has been used successfully to treat individuals with mild and moderate levels of ID. Some modifications include:
- Using language that the individual can understand;
- Awareness of the developmental level of the individual;
- Making interpretations appropriate to the developmental level, cognitive level, and knowledge base of the individual;
- An understanding of the possible life experiences of an individual with ID (see Chapter 1), and
- Observations of the individual in his or her environment as well as frequent contact with caregivers (Ruth 2001).

Example: Psychodynamically Oriented Psychotherapy

J.'s history of explosive behavior indicated they were frequently exhibited when she was in situations where she had minimal options and choices. The therapist helped her discuss current situations in which she became explosive—swearing, yelling, and hitting others. As therapy progressed, J. became more secure and trusting with the therapeutic relationship. She was then able to report experiencing intense feelings of anger, frustration, and rage during these episodes. She began to demonstrate an increased ability to articulate current conflicts as well as her thoughts and feelings associated with them. The therapist then helped her discuss past conflicts followed by informed interpretations (ideas the therapist developed from his or her training, from all of the information gathered by history and information from the sessions). J. came to recognize that these were experiences where she felt she had little control over her life. She was then able to uncover and trace her feelings of grief, anger, and shame to surgery involving a tubal-ligation. She had felt coerced into consenting to it by her guardian. She was able to relate these unresolved feelings with current behaviors when she was in situations that elicited similar feelings. J.'s courage to address this unresolved grief, associated feelings, and the anxiety that they produced enabled her to develop control of her behavior outbursts.

Supportive Therapy

Supportive therapy is a relationship-oriented approach to treatment. This modality is effective in treating individuals who have experienced a period of regression due to some stressful event. The ultimate goal of this treatment is to help restore the individual to the previous level of functioning. Individuals in this regressed state are often overcome by feelings of anxiety, rejection, and fears that interfere with their ability to use coping strategies that they had once utilized.

In this type of therapy the therapist assumes a much more active role in providing guidance for the client to talk about his or her distress and problems and attempts to help him or her make successful decisions. Whenever possible the individual is also helped to become more self-aware.

Some commonly used interventions include:
- Assisting the client decrease external stressors by changing the environment or temporarily increasing the support and attention given by the caregivers;
- Development of leisure time and pleasurable activities and arranging for caregivers to assist in making this occur;
- Doing whatever is needed to help the client feel more secure and accepted, both in the therapy sessions and in home and day programs;
- Temporarily meeting the dependency needs of the individual such as calling for the cab at the end of the session;
- Providing guidance and recommendations for dealing with current conflicts, problems, and stressful issues;
- Assisting individuals to verbalize unexpressed strong emotions to provide relief of overwhelming depression and anxiety, and
- Strengthen coping strategies (Kaplan & Sadock 1991).

Example: Supportive Therapy

M. is a 35-year-old woman with mild ID and a mood disorder. She had experienced a variety of levels of residential living from community residences to supervised apartments. She had work placements in sheltered workshops, work enclaves, and supportive work in competitive employment. M. was not able to sustain her least restrictive levels of placements. In these settings she became increasingly anxious, experienced decreased self-esteem and confidence, and developed an increase in paranoid thinking. In therapy her comments suggested a hypersensitivity to others, a fear of failure, and a sense of rejection. In addition to medication adjustments, she required increased reality testing (help recognizing real things from imagined things) to decrease these thoughts and fears, increased support by frequent reassurances that she was doing well, and guidance with problem-solving and working out interpersonal relationships.

Over time, M. has been able to develop a positive, more open relationship with the therapist, and she is beginning to generalize this. She is able to "check out" with others when she is experiencing a feeling of rejection or disapproval by doing things like asking them if she has done something to upset them. She is gradually working toward her goal of increasing her independence and returning to the least restrictive level possible.

Dialectical Behavioral Therapy

This treatment modality was specifically developed and designed by Marsha Linehan (1993) for the treatment of Borderline Personality Disorder (BPD). It is based on several theories including, cognitive behavioral theory for its focus on change, Zen for its focus on acceptance, and Dialectics for its focus on acceptance and change. In this model the etiology of BPD is based on a biosocial theory that makes two major assumptions: there is a biological dysfunction in the person's emotional regulation system and a chronic exposure to an invalidating environment. This combination leads to the pervasive emotional dysregulation that individuals with BPD exhibit.

The skills training program of Dialectical Behavioral Therapy (DBT) focuses on four skills modules to "learn and refine skills in changing behavioral, emotional, and thinking patterns associated with problems in living that are causing misery and distress" (Linehan, 1993).

They are:
- Mindfulness skills, meaning staying focused on what is going on at the moment and experiencing it without judgement, which are targeted to decrease identity confusion, feelings of emptiness, and cognitive deregulation;
- Interpersonal skills that are designed to decrease interpersonal chaos and fears of abandonment;
- Emotional regulation skills that focus on decreasing labile affect and excessive anger, and
- Distress tolerance skills that assist individuals with decreasing impulsive behaviors, suicide threats, and parasuicidal behaviors.

Linehan has developed a skills manual with training material for each skills module completed that includes lecture material, handouts, and homework assignments. A manual has not yet been published for individuals with ID and BPD, but one is in the process of being developed. Some of the modifications that have been used in practice to adapt this material to the learning style and needs of individuals with ID include:
- Limiting sessions to 45 minutes or 1 hour verses 2 or 2 1/2 hours;
- Increasing the number of sessions spent on each skill module to ensure internalization of new material;
- Giving more homework assignments to help reinforce skill acquisition;
- Using more active mindful exercises, that is, using more game type activities;
- Using more role-playing activities;
- Training day and residential staff, including having caregivers from all settings participate in training of all four modules, and
- Simplifying diary cards, using homework assignments with more concrete language, shortening explanations, and using pictures or clip art on handouts and homework assignments.

GROUP THERAPY

The history of group therapy began in the 1950s as an intervention to assist individuals with emotional stress by providing support and education. Since then, group therapy has been an effective treatment modality for individuals with ID.

Individuals with ID often must cope with feelings of rejection, exclusion, decreased sense of self worth, and superficial peer relationships. Fletcher (1984) reported that group therapy could increase an individual's sense of security, trust, and community, which can in turn assist in decreasing emotional stress. Additional benefits of group therapy include:

- Improved peer relationships;
- Increased problem-solving skills;
- Improved listening skills;
- Increased ability to disclose issues and feelings;
- Improved social skills;
- Acceptance of ID;
- A sense of empowerment and independence;
- Development of assertiveness skills, and
- Improved anger-management skills (Fletcher 1984).

The unique aspect of group therapy is that it allows individuals to obtain support from their peers who are experiencing similar issues, problems, and concerns. This exchange between individuals can have a dramatic impact on decreasing an individual's sense of isolation, increasing self-esteem, and assisting with achievement of goals. Lindenbaum and Lindenbaum-Cox (1993) reported the following as commonly discussed themes in group sessions:

- Environmental stressors;
- Inappropriate behaviors;
- Coping with ID;
- Desires to increase independence;
- Separation/individuation issues;
- Sexual issues, and
- Family/system dynamics.

Some common activities in group sessions that are useful tools to assist individuals with ID to address issues include:

- Role-playing;
- Modeling;
- Relaxation exercises, and
- Self-esteem games/activities, for example, listing strengths, celebrating successes.

The therapist's role and skills have a significant impact on developing a milieu that provides a safe and trusting environment and facilitates client growth. As in any group, three stages of development are necessary. The first phase focuses on goal setting, orientation, and the development of group identity. Frequently, group members will demonstrate an increased dependence on the group therapist at this stage and require prompts and redirection to engage with group members. The second stage is characterized by exploration and testing of the group leader and conflict among group members. Individuals may verbalize resistance and/or drop out at this stage, if conflicts are not addressed. It is helpful to maintain contact with caregivers, particularly at this stage, to support continuation in group therapy. The third stage leads to the development of a cohesive unit where there is a sense of mutual support, trust, and improved peer interactions.

It is important that the group therapist possesses a caring, genuine, and empathetic style that encourages interaction and expression among group members. The therapist's role is multifaceted. It includes functioning as a role model, teacher, facilitator, and therapist. Therapists frequently need to take a more active and directive approach than might occur in a non-ID group.

Groups comprised of individuals with mild ID often function well with an open-ended, client-centered approach. The therapist needs to facilitate discussion, encourage sharing, and assist the group in giving praise, encouragement, and feedback to each other. Clarification, support, and interpretation can be useful and effective treatment interventions.

Individuals with moderate, severe, and profound ID often respond more positively to groups that are more structured and directive. The therapist functions more in the role of instructor and role model. The use of social skills games, anger-management programs, and role-playing has been effective in providing the necessary structure and helpful teaching.

Various individual treatment modalities can be adapted and utilized in groups such as relationship therapy, transactional analysis, and rational emotive therapy. Tomasulo (2000) has developed a model that adapts Interactive Behavior Therapy to treat individuals with ID.

Quoting several individuals who participate in group therapy best expresses its benefits:
"Group helps me talk about my problems."
"Helps me feel good, have good behavior."
"Brings out all the stuff I keep inside."
"Helps me decide what to do about things."
"I feel good when I get feedback from others because then I know they are listening and they understand." (List, 1999)

Systemic Therapy

No one lives in a vacuum. There is a large network of people who are more or less closely involved in an individual's life. For someone with ID these people generally have a great deal of influence in all aspects of his or her life. The caregivers have a much greater impact on an individual with ID than any therapist can. System theory teaches us that changing something in one part of the system causes a reaction in other parts of the system. Thus, with individuals who are dependent upon and influenced by their caregivers, therapy must often include the whole system.

Without a unified approach, individual caregivers may attempt to resolve issues independently, using different and conflicting interventions. This can lead to an increase or worsening of the individual's symptoms, blaming among care providers, and eventually burnout for all. An initial assessment is needed to understand how each component of the system—day program staff, teachers, parents, client, and any other care providers—understands the client and thinks about the problem, including how they interact with one another. This may be accomplished through interviews and direct observations in the settings where the individual lives, plays, and works. It is important to have an understanding of the strengths, resources, problems, and conflicts of all of the individuals and various components of the system. Some additional information to obtain during the assessment process include:

- How individual and caregivers define the problems/concerns;
- How individual and caregivers perceive the cause of problems/concerns;
- Strengths and weaknesses of individual, environment, caregivers;
- Current coping strategies; are they effective or maladaptive;
- Is there collaboration among caregivers;
- Is there consistency in addressing issues with individual and caregivers;
- Is the environment supportive or punitive;
- Is there stability in the environment or are there frequent changes in routine or turnover of staff, and
- What are the caregivers' attitudes toward the individual?

Utilizing a systems approach as part of treatment can be effective and provide assistance on a variety of levels (Rotthaus, 2001). At the individual level, it can help provide a better understanding of how environmental stresses, changes, and pressures may be contributing to the symptoms. Behavioral skills to assist the individual with symptom control are often best addressed utilizing this approach. For new skill development to be learned and generalized to all environmental settings, consistent and frequent rehearsals as well as positive feedback are crucial. A systems' approach allows for this consistency and reinforcement, leading to more successful and long-lasting behavioral changes.

At the caregiver level, consistency and improved communication can be major benefits. Increased support and trust among caregivers can be developed through the use of feedback, encouragement, troubleshooting, and validation of feelings (Nezu, Nezu, & Gill-Weiss, 1992). Regular meetings with the therapist and caregivers are helpful to: reach consensus on identified problem areas, prioritize which problems and symptoms to address, create a treatment plan for identified issues, and develop a system to monitor and evaluate the effectiveness of the treatment plan.

The partnerships that are developed and the effectiveness of problem-solving strategies using a systems approach are beneficial not only for the individual with ID but also for all involved in their care. In fact, it is often essential to enable individuals to be successfully integrated in all aspects of their lives: family, day program, residential program, recreational program, and community (Nezu et al., 1992).

Family Therapy

At times the family may need their own therapy. In fact, family therapy may be helpful throughout the lifecycle to give the family support in dealing with the stressors produced by having a child with an ID. (See stresses noted above and in Chapter 1.)

Initially grieving the loss of a normal child may be facilitated by couple therapy. Then as the child ages, family therapy can facilitate communication among the family members. Where dysfunctional interactions have developed, family therapy can help families make effective modifications. It can be useful in helping families recognize the benefits of fostering as much independence as possible in their family member with the disability. It can support the parents and siblings in accepting and encouraging the individual to make steps towards independence. Group family therapy has been successful in helping families learn to verbalize and share feelings (Szymanski & Kiernan, 1983). Shame and embarrassment are two emotions often felt by the family of an individual with ID and can lead to isolation (Rotthaus 2001). Group therapy with other families may be the first step away from isolation and a move to more healthy ways of functioning. There are a variety of models of family therapy, for example, Bowen, Satir, and Minuchin, to name a few. All of the major models have slightly different interventions, but the overall goals are generally the same. The major goals of family therapy include:

- Resolve or decrease conflicts within the family;
- Increase understanding of individual family member's needs;
- Encourage age appropriate relationships;
- Strengthen coping strategies, and
- Enhance family values that encourage healthy growth and development. (Kaplan & Sadock 1991)

All of these goals are valid with families with or without a family member with ID. Characteristics that foster positive family relationships include:

- Establishment of clear boundaries;
- Flexibility;
- Clear rules;
- Consistent enforcement of rules;
- Expressions of positive regard;
- Honest and clear communication patterns, and
- Reinforcement of adaptive behaviors.

SUMMARY

The diagnosis and treatment of individuals with ID and mental disorders is an ongoing and evolving process. Significant progress has been made in the past 10 to 15 years in terms of recognizing, diagnosing, and treating mental disorders in this population.

Individuals with ID and mental disorders are able to benefit from traditional modalities of psychotherapy. Often only simple modifications are needed to enhance the effectiveness of the therapy. As in the general population, these therapies can be used solely or in combination with each other.

For successful and sustained changes to occur as a result of psychotherapy, a multifaceted approach is frequently indicated. In addition to individual therapy, many individuals with ID benefit from group therapy, family therapy, and systemic approaches. It is imperative that therapists working with individuals with ID have an understanding of ID and the skills and abilities of the individual to develop strong, warm, empathetic therapeutic relationships.

TABLE 7.1
Types of Individual Therapy With Modifications

Type	Goal	Modifications
Transactional Analysis	Help the individual look at his or her behavior, identify the appropriate ego states, and make decisions to think and behave in the adult mode, which will improve self-esteem and level of independence.	Educate patient regarding the 3 ego states with simplified and concrete language geared to their cognitive level, role playing can be helpful
		Clear, concise examples of individual's behavior exemplifying the 3 ego states need to be done in an ongoing basis
		Use of role playing to practice changing behaviors and interactions with others
		Collaborated with care provides to assist with practicing role plays outside the therapy sessions to facilitate generalization of new skills in all environmental settings
Behavior Therapy	Change of maladaptive behaviors without insight into underlying causes.	Include the individual in the treatment planning
		Choose a target behavior to reinforce
		Select an appropriate reinforcer
		Ensure that the individual understands the behavior that is being reinforced
		Implement the program
Cognitive Behavioral Therapy	Identify and change distorted thoughts that maintain symptoms. Focuses on changing current behaviors by changing thoughts that are connected to these behaviors.	Increase length of treatment, 1-2 years may be needed to achieve goals
		Collaborate with staff and family members to assist patient and therapist identify distorted/irrational thoughts
		Enlist assistance from caregivers to assist patient with completion of homework assignments, e.g. rehearsing new responses via role playing
		Build in positive reinforcement for completion of homework
Dialectical Behavioral Therapy	Focuses on 4 skills modules to "learn and refine skills in changing behavioral, emotional and thinking patterns associated with problems in living that are causing misery and distress"	Limiting sessions to 45 minutes or one hour verses 2 or 2 ½ hours
		Increasing the number of sessions spent on each skill module to ensure internalization of new material
		Giving more homework assignments to help reinforce skill acquisition
		Using more active mindful exercises, i.e. using more game type activities
		Using more role playing activities
		Training day and residential staff. This includes having caregivers from all settings participate in training of all 4 modules
		Simplifying diary cards, using homework assignments with more concrete; language, shortening explanations and using pictures or clip art on handouts and homework assignments.
Psychodynamically Oriented Psychotherapy	To connect past, usually unconscious experiences with present behaviors and change them.	Language is needed to ensure that the individual can understand the ideas the therapist is discussing
		Awareness of the developmental level of the client is needed to help make appropriate interpretations and to understand the possible life experiences of an individual with ID
		An observation of an individual in his or her environment as well as frequent contact with caregivers is also important

REFERENCES

Beck, J. (1995). *Cognitive therapy*. New York: The Guilford Press.

Cobb, H. (1973). *Citizen advocacy and the rights of the handicapped: Citizen advocacy* (pp. 149-160). Toronto, Ontario, Canada: The National Institute on Mental Retardation.

Fletcher, R. (1984). Group therapy with mentally retarded persons with emotional disorders. *Psychiatric Aspects of Mental Retardation Reviews, 3,* 21-24.

Harris, T. (1973). *I'm OK-You're OK*. New York: Harper & Row.

Hurley, A. & Sovner, R. (1986). Behavior Modification IV: Positive reinforcement. *Psychiatric Aspects of Mental Retardation Reviews, 5,* 57-62.

Judge, C. (1983). Self-awareness of mentally retarded persons. *Psychiatric Aspects of Mental Retardation Newsletter, 2,* 42-43.

Kaplan, H. & Sadock, B. (1991). *Synopsis of psychiatry*. Baltimore: Williams and Wilkins Co.

Keller, E. (2000). Points of intervention: Facilitating the process of psychotherapy with people who have developmental disability. In R. Fletcher (Ed.), *Therapy approaches for persons with mental retardation* (pp. 27-45). Kingston, NY: NADD Press.

Laterza, P. (1983). *An eclectic approach to group work with the mentally retarded: Differential diagnosis and treatment in social work* (pp. 520-529). New York: The Free Press.

Levitas, A. & Gilson, S. (1987). Psychosocial crisis in the lives of mentally retarded people. *Psychiatric Aspects of Mentally Retardation Reviews, 6,* 27-31.

Levitas, A. & Gilson, S. F. (1994) Psychosocial Development of Children and Adolescents with Mild Mental Retardation. In N. Bouras (Ed.), *Mental health in mental retardation*. London: Cambridge University Press.

Lindenbaum, L., & Lindenbaum-Cox, D. (Speakers) (1993). *Group therapy: Theoretical and practical applications in the treatment of the dually diagnosed.* (Audio CD Recording No. CT93-301C). Kingston, NY: NADD

Linehan, M. (1993). *Skills training manual for treating borderline personality disorders*. New York: The Guilford Press.

List, A. (1999). *The Effectiveness of Therapy Groups for Clients with Dual Diagnosis. Junior BSW Research Project*. Rochester, NY: Nazareth College

Nezu, C., Nezu, A., & Gill-Weiss, M. (1992). *Psychopathology in persons with mental retardation*. Champaign, IL: Research Press Company.

Nirje, B. (1969). The normalization principle and its human management implications. In R. Kugel & W. Wolfensberger (Eds.). *Changing patterns in residential services for the mentally retarded.* Washington, DC: President's Committee on Mental Retardation.

Rotthaus, W. (2001). Systemic therapy. In A. Dosen & K. Day (Eds.). *Treating mental illness and behavior disorders in children and adults with mental retardation*. Washington, DC: American Psychiatric Press, Inc.

Ruth, R. (2001). Psychoanalytic Therapies. In A. Dosen & K. Day (Eds.), *Treating Mental Illbess and Behavioral Disorders in Children and Adults with Mental Retardation (pp. 133-143)*. Washington, DC: American Psychiatric Press.

Sovner, R., & Hurley, A. (1983). The subjective experience. *Psychiatric Aspects of Mental Retardation Newsletter, 2,* 42-43.

Szymanski, L.S. & Kiernan, W. E. (1983). Multiple family group therapy with developmentally disabled adolescents and young adults. *International Journal of Group Psychotherapy 33,* 521-534.

Tomasulo, Daniel. (2000). Group Therapy for People with Mental Retardation. *Therapy Approaches for Persons with Mental Retardation*. Kingston, NY: NADD Press 65-83.

8

Applied Behavior Analysis
Peter Sturmey, Howie Reyer, Ronald Lee and Adrienne Robek

INTRODUCTION

From the 1930s through the 1950s, B. F. Skinner and his colleagues conducted a series of learning studies using pigeons and rats. These studies showed that behavior was related to the current environment as well as the animals' learning history. As seen in Box 8.1, Skinner distinguished between his operant conditioning model and Pavlov's classical conditioning model.

The effectiveness of behavior analytic technologies has also been demonstrated with humans. Fuller (1949) increased the rate of arm-raising in a person with ID and multiple disabilities using warm, sweet milk as a reinforcer. Greenspoon (1955) demonstrated that he could increase the rate of an undergraduate's use of adjectives by using contingent social approval. Ayllon & Michael (1959) showed that teaching staff that used reinforcement to increase the rate of self-help, talking, and vocational skills could vastly improve the behavior of individuals in a psychiatric hospital. A variety of behavior-reduction procedures were also developed to decrease the rate of delusional talk, refusal to eat, and aggression. By the mid-1960s, there were demonstrations of the use of Applied Behavior Analysis (ABA) to a wide range of practical problems in clinical and educational settings.

The ABA model was further strengthened by demonstrations that behavior disturbances

---

BOX 8.1
PAVLOVIAN AND SKINNERIAN MODELS

Pavlov's Classical Conditioning Model
When a dog is given food (an unconditioned stimulus), it salivates (an unconditioned response). If the dog's owner rings a bell (conditioned stimulus) every time that the dog is given food, eventually every time that the bell rings, it will begin to salivate (a conditioned response), even in the absence of food.

Skinner's Operant Conditioning Model
Both humans and other animals exhibit many behaviors. Certain forms of behavior will be selected by the environment through reinforcement and extinction. Behaviors that are reinforced by food, other people, or other stimuli will increase in frequency and be strengthened. Other behaviors that are not reinforced will be weakened, reduced in frequency, and eventually extinguished.

could result *exclusively* from learning, rather than intra-psychic conflict, brain damage, dysregulation of neurotransmitters, or mental disorder. For example, Schaefer (1970) shaped self-injurious behavior (SIB) in two Rhesus monkeys. During early shaping sessions, every time that the monkey raised its arm, it was given a pellet of food. Within 12 minutes, the first monkey had been taught to raise its paw above its head and then touch its head. The monkey's behavior was then brought under the stimulus control of the experimenter's own social behavior. This was accomplished by reinforcing SIB only when it occurred after the experimenter said the phrase, "poor boy…" Reinforcement was not delivered for SIB when the experimenter said nothing. As a result, the monkey learned to touch his head only when the experimenter's behavior signaled the availability of reinforcement for that behavior. Schaefer (1970) replicated these results with another monkey. He taught a third monkey to bang the cage wall with its paw, and then, ultimately, to bang its head against the cage wall with increasing speed. This study demonstrated that pathological behaviors could be the result of learning. It further demonstrated that learned pathological behaviors could also come under the control of the social behavior of other people. Haughton & Ayllon (1998) demonstrated that unusual human behavior could also be learned. (See Box 8.2.)

BOX 8.2
EXAMPLE OF BIZARRE BEHAVIOR ACCOUNTED FOR BY LEARNING ALONE

Can the learning model account for human psychopathology? Haughton & Ayllon (1998) conducted a study in which a 54-year-old client with schizophrenia was the participant. Hospital staff described that she refused to do anything except smoke. Baseline data showed that 80% of her time was spent sitting, lying in bed, or walking. During the baseline, she was given only one cigarette at each meal. As a result, cigarettes became powerful reinforcers. To develop a novel class of behavior, an arbitrary response was selected – holding a broom. This response was then reinforced with cigarettes. In a few days, she paced the room while holding the broom. Additionally, if others attempted to take the broom away from her, she resisted firmly and, occasionally, with aggression. Her broom-holding was characteristic of behavior typically described as being "compulsive." Two psychiatrists were then asked to evaluate her behavior. One psychiatrist explained her behavior as "…a stereotyped form of behavior such as is commonly seen in rather regressed schizophrenics and is rather analogous to the way small children or infants refuse to be parted from some favorite toy, piece of rag, etc." The second psychiatrist gave an explanation which concluded that the broom could represent either "(1) a child that gives her love, and she gives him in return her devotion, (2) a phallic symbol, or (3) the scepter of an omnipotent queen." Thus, it is possible that behavior disturbances can be shaped in humans. When people, including mental health professionals, are unaware of a person's learning history, they are likely to ascribe the causes of behavior to mysterious, unobservable causes, such as mental disorders or regression.

Basic ABA concepts

The field of ABA resulted from a combination of the applications of Skinner's operant psychology, operant models of maladaptive behaviors, and social concern to improve human behavior. The aim of ABA is to change a person's behavioral repertoire to include many adaptive skills and appropriate behaviors that enable the person to be effective and to show behaviors that are valued by themselves, their significant others, and society. ABA is very specific in how language is used. Terms are used with very particular meanings that can be a little different from everyday use. Some commonly used terms are defined in Box 8.3.

Baer, Wolf, & Risley (1968) defined six characteristics of ABA that distinguish it from other approaches. First, it is applied; that is, it focuses on behaviors that are socially important. Thus, the behavior studies must be important to the person studied, the important people around them, and to society. Second, ABA is behavioral; behavioral means measuring and changing what people do. ABA is disinterested in reports from staff or family members in clinics or meetings: they are often inaccurate and invalid. Instead, ABA goes out into the natural environment and both observes and measures the behavior of interest there. Third, ABA is also analytic; ABA is not merely interested in changing behavior. It is also interested in understanding the learning mechanisms that cause that change. Baer and others said, "We have analyzed a behavior when we can turn the behavior on and off". This is done by directly manipulating the environmental variables that affect that behavior. Fourth, ABA is technological; the procedures used in ABA are precisely defined. In this way we can be sure of what the treatment was, and others can replicate the treatment with confidence. Thus, "The treatment consisted of reinforcement" is not an adequate and technological description of treatment. However, if we say "Each time John said 'hi'

BOX 8.3
SOME DEFINTIONS OF IMPORTANT BEHAVIORAL TERMS

Behavior
Skinner (1938/1999) defines "behavior as any action by an organism that has a measurable effect on the environment …".

Reinforcer
"To reinforce means to make stronger or more pronounced. In operant conditioning, reinforcement is a process whereby a consequence strengthens the behavior on which it is contingent … reflected in its increased frequency, duration or magnitude. " (Sarfino, 2001, p.111.)

Antecedent
"Cues that precede and set the occasion for particular behaviors" (Sarafino, 2001, p. 421.)

Functional analysis
"An experimenter has achieved an analysis of a behavior when he can exercise control over it … an ability of the experimenter to turn the behavior on and off or up and down at will." (Baer et al., 1968, p. 94.)

the peer smiled and said 'hi' within 2 seconds," then we have a technologically adequate definition of our treatment. Fifth, ABA interventions have conceptual integrity; this means that there is a clear description of the learning mechanisms that are believed to account for behavior change. For example, we would not only say "John's whining was ignored." Rather, we would also say, "John's whining was placed on attention-extinction." Finally, treatments based on ABA should be effective. They should produce effects that are large and meaningful for each particular individual. Many other treatments focus on the average scores of groups and statistical significance. Such an approach ignores how important the change is and the importance of the change for each individual.

ABA Has A Strong Evidence Base

Interventions based on ABA have very strong scientific support. For example, Didden, Duker, & Korzilius, (1997) conducted a systematic analysis of 482 empirical behavior analytic studies that involved participants with ID. There were 1,451 comparisons between baselines and treatments. In order to compare different interventions, behavioral procedures were broken down into different types of procedures. One class of intervention was response-contingent procedures. These were procedures based on reinforcement for the absence of the maladaptive response or punishment of the target response. Another class of intervention was response-noncontingent procedures. These were defined as procedures such as stimulation, environmental enrichment, and non-contingent reinforcement. A final class of procedures included those based on antecedent control. Interventions based on antecedent control modify events that occur before the target behavior. For example, stimuli that provoke the maladaptive behavior might be removed, and stimuli that make appropriate behavior more likely are introduced.

Didden and others found that response-contingent procedures were more effective than other approaches such as antecedent-control procedures, pharmacological interventions, or response-noncontingent procedures. Combined treatment-packages of procedures that included both reinforcement and prompts were found to be superior to single-component behavioral procedures. Functional assessments and the more precise methods used in functional analyses, which systematically manipulate environmental variables to determine their effects on behavior, were associated with larger effect sizes.

Instructional and treatment procedures based on the principles of ABA have been endorsed as highly effective means for increasing appropriate responding and reducing a wide range of behavioral disturbances (Expert Consensus Panel, 2000; NYSDH, 1999; Surgeon General, 2000). Interventions using the framework of ABA are based on a model that assumes that many behaviors, including behavioral disturbances and symptoms of mental disorders, are learned or have a significant learning component to them. ABA emphasizes the analysis of specific aspects of each individual's current environment, their learning history, and the interaction between the two. For example, one person's aggression might be reinforced by attention, whereas another person's aggression might be reinforced by escape from difficult tasks. Thus, interventions should be developed only after an understanding of the nature of the interaction between that person's behavior and his/her environment has been achieved. Finally, interventions based on ABA are considered positive to the extent that they focus on teaching functional skills to replace, rather than to suppress, undesirable behaviors, and that they directly improve that person's quality of life.

These findings have important implications for current practice. ABA should be the intervention of choice, since it has the strongest evidence base supporting its use. Interventions based on ABA should be based on a functional assessment and should be multi-component packages of both response-contingent procedures, rather than response non-contingent procedures, and should include antecedents.

METHODS OF APPLIED BEHAVIOR ANALYSIS

ABA incorporates many methods for data collection. Initially, these may include interviews and questionnaires. Eventually, direct observation in the natural environment, and, ultimately, experimental analyses of the behavior are conducted. Often, these methods are combined following procedural guidelines. O'Neill, Horner, Albin, Sprague, Storey, & Newton (1997) describe a set of procedural guidelines that are often used. These include structured interviews, procedures for collecting direct observational data, manipulating variables that might influence behavior and procedures for writing behavior support plans.

Interviews

A common way of collecting information is by assessment interviews. ABA often uses a specific form of assessment interview referred to as semi-structured behavioral interviewing (O'Neill et al., 1997; Sturmey, 1996). In semi-structured interviewing, topics such as the presenting problem, the client's history and current strengths, and their goals for change are covered. Typically each section or subsection of an interview begins with an open-ended remark, such as, "Tell me about the problem." Open-ended questions and remarks solicit a wide range of material but may also result in indirect and/or disorganized answers. After several open-ended questions are asked, closed-ended questions are used to clarify specific points. An example of such a question is, "Does it happen more at work or at home?" Summary statements are used to check for accuracy and to solicit further information. Conducting effective semi-structured behavioral interviews is a skill that requires training that consists of, but is not limited to, observation of and feedback to the interviewer by a mentor or other supervisor. Interviews can be conducted with a variety of informants who know the client well, including family members, peers and staff, and, in some cases, clients themselves. Specific interview protocols are described in O'Neill et al., (1997).

Questionnaires

Questionnaires can be used to assess both the form and function of disturbed behaviors. Questionnaires that measure the form of a response are empirically based and refer to specific behaviors such as "hits others," "screams," and so on. Other questionnaires are based on DSM-IV-TR (APA, 2000) or other psychiatric classification schemes. They often use scales that correspond to specific mental disorders. In these questionnaires, items are defined as clearly as possible and then rated based on frequency, intensity, or severity. The Diagnostic Assessment for the Severely Handicapped II (Matson et al., 1996) is a measure based on DSM-IV and was designed specifically for adult persons with severe or profound ID. Other measures focus purely on the client's observable behavior rather than any possible mental disorder. For example, the Aberrant Behavior Checklist (Singh, Aman, & Turbott, 1985) is a good example of a measure based on observable behavior rather than specific psychiatric symptoms. These measures can be useful as an initial screening, for example, when a new client is first referred. They can also provide some guidance as to the maladaptive responses that should be addressed through intervention or psychiatric diagnosis. Nevertheless, they should be regarded as general screens that should be supplemented by other assessment procedures and should not be used alone. A trained professional, such as a psychologist, usually administers and scores the questionnaires. As with interviews, a wide variety of people who know the client well can provide information.

Questionnaires have also been used to measure the function of behavior. For example, the Motivation Assessment Scale (Durand & Crimmins, 1986) assesses the extent to which a specific form of behavior is maintained by attention, escape from demands, access to tangible items, or automatic reinforcement (i.e., internal or self-stimulation). There are a variety of such scales available, and they can be a useful part of an initial evaluation to assess the function of behavior. Nevertheless, many scales have been assembled on the basis of intuition and lack essential psychometric properties such as reliability. Thus, questionnaires that are designed to assess the function of a response should be used cautiously.

Direct Observation

The method that is most characteristic of ABA is direct observation of behavior. Behavior has specific physical dimensions. These include frequency, rate, duration, and intensity. Behavior also produces permanent products such as number of words typed or weight of garbage. Often, the behavior of any individual is orderly, sequenced, and closely related to and influenced by the environment. The environment includes temporally proximal stimuli such as antecedents and consequences. Antecedents are events that occur close in time to the behavior of interest. Antecedents can include requests from others to do something, the removal of a preferred item, and so on. Consequences can include the presentation of a stimulus, for example, a nurse applying a bandage, or removal of a stimulus, such as a staff member removing a noisily boisterous peer. Additionally, the environment also includes distal stimuli, such as deprivation and satiation. For example, if a student has eaten 30 minutes ago then food is unlikely to be an effective reinforcer. Likewise, if no one has talked to a student for 90 minutes then the student might work well for praise. The frequency of a response is measured by recording the number of instances of it. The rate is obtained by dividing the frequency by the duration of the observation. Duration can be measured directly using stopwatches or by writing down the beginning and end of each target behavior. Duration can also be estimated using various time-sampling methods. For example, an observer might note once every minute throughout the day if a person is working at exactly that moment. Direct observation, ABC charts, and narrative descriptions of the antecedent, behavior, and consequence for each instance of the target response are used to describe the relationship between the behavior of interest and the environment. Scatterplots, a grid of the day and time of day, can be used to examine the relation between the environment and behavior (Touchette, MacDonald, & Langer, 1985).

Experimental Functional Analyses

Identification of the environmental factors that motivate and maintain each client's disturbed behavior is critical for developing an intervention with the highest probability of success. One of the purposes of the experimental analyses of behavior is to design individually tailored, effective interventions. Experimental analyses of behavior involve the systematic and deliberate manipulations of variables by the experimenter or clinician. For example, a clinician might deliberately compare a clients' behavior when an easy task is presented with the client's behavior when a difficult task is presented. Wacker, Berg, Harding, Derby, Asmus, & Healy, (1998) illustrate the use of a functional analysis with children with ID. Each parent was provided with a treatment plan that involved functional communication training (FCT). FCT involves teaching the child a communicative response to replace his/her disturbed behavior. For example, the children were taught to sign, "Please" to obtain attention or "Break" to obtain a brief escape from tasks. The children learned the communication skills, and subsequently their disturbed behaviors reduced. Also, there were other changes in behavior that were rated positively by other people who knew the children well. These findings supported the use of functional analyses for the purpose of developing an intervention matched to the results of the analysis.

APPLICATIONS TO MENTAL DISORDERS AND INTELLECTUAL DISABILITIES: CASE EXAMPLES

Psychotic Speech

Durand & Crimmins, (1987) determined the function of psychotic speech in a child with autism. The first of three experiments analyzed the role of adult attention during easy tasks and difficult tasks. During baseline, the subject worked on the easy task with one-to-one adult attention. Correct responses were praised and incorrect responses were followed by, "No that's not right." During *Decreased Attention* there was a reduced rate of adult attention with the same easy task. During *Increased Task Difficulty* there was one-to-one adult attention throughout the difficult task. The results showed low mean rates of psychotic speech in both baseline and *Decreased Attention*. During *Increased Task Difficulty* the rate of psychotic speech systematically increased. This indicated that psychotic speech might function to escape task demands.

Experiment Two used time-out from attention and tasks (i.e., 10-second head-turn and removal of task materials). The data also supported an escape hypothesis. Almost half of these sessions were spent in time-out and the proportion of psychotic speech during the time-in periods was much greater. Since psychotic speech functioned to terminate task demands, Experiment Three provided an alternative means of escape in order to reduce the frequency of psychotic speech. The child was taught to say, "Help me." If this request was followed by teacher assistance, it should reduce the task difficulty. During the *Help me* condition the mean rate of psychotic speech systematically declined to low levels. Thus, this study identified the function of psychotic speech and treated it by teaching an appropriate communicative response that served the same function as psychotic speech.

Depression

Lindsay, Howells, & Pitcaithly, (1993) used a simplified method of cognitive therapy in two adults with mild ID one of whom exhibited frequent suicidal thoughts and threats. They taught the clients to learn the relationships between their thoughts, feelings, and behavior using both role-play and live practice. For both participants ratings of depression declined after treatment and were maintained at follow-up six weeks later. For the client who was suicidal, the frequency of suicidal statements declined from 40 recorded in *one* hour in the first assessment to zero, 12 weeks later.

Matson, (1982) treated the behavioral characteristics associated with depression, such as the number of words spoken, somatic complaints, irritability, lack of grooming, negative self-statements, flat affect, eye contact, and speech latency in four adults with ID. They were asked questions each weekday that were specific to both somatic complaints and negative self-statements. Treatment consisted of 10 to 35 sessions of reinforcing appropriate responses such as eye contact and social interaction with tokens, by instruction, performance feedback, modeling, and role-playing. After treatment, the behavioral characteristics of depression declined in all four clients. Further, the results were maintained from four to six months and were also reflected on two general measures of depression.

Sturmey, (1995) evaluated the use of 24-hour social isolation as a treatment for repeated suicidal threats with a man with moderate ID, multiple psychiatric diagnoses, and acting-out behaviors. His threats resulted in multiple transfers to the state hospital. It appeared that his threats were maintained by attention, including access to multiple nurses as well as the medical director, admission to the infirmary, transfer to the state hospital, and so on. He was first referred when he began making suicidal threats on the same day that he returned from a stay at the state hospital. His interdisciplinary team identified that this pattern of admission had completely disrupted any programming for this man for over a year. To design an intervention based on this hypothesis, a suicide watch was developed that minimized access to attention. This included placement in a quiet room without access to TV, other people, or any other potential reinforcers. Meals were served in that room. Staff members were trained to stay just outside the room and observe but not to talk to him. This procedure led to restitution of programming and virtual elimination of suicide threats within three months.

These studies suggest that behavior characteristic of mood disorder, just like other behavior, can be observed and modified based on an analysis of their relation to environmental events, which can be manipulated. Likewise, intervention plans for suicidal behavior can also be developed based on functional assessment information.

Obsessive-Compulsive Disorder

Formulations of compulsive behavior have traditionally emphasized the role of negative reinforcement. It is often assumed that rituals serve to either escape or avoid anxiety. Although treatments based on this analysis, such as systematic desensitization, have had considerable success, an analysis of individual differences is essential for treatment development. Rincover, Newsom, & Carr, (1979) investigated the role of two possible forms of sensory reinforcement in two children who engaged in a high frequency of compulsive light-switching. The sensory consequences maintaining light-switching might be either changes in illumination or the clicking sound of the light switch. Therefore, two forms of sensory extinction procedures were designed, one for each of the two sensory consequences of light-switching. In the first form of sensory extinction, light-switching did not produce a change in illumination. In the second form of sensory extinction, the clicking sound of the light switch was eliminated (i.e., the light still came on, but there was no clicking sound). For the first child, when switch operation no longer produced illumination changes, switching systematically decreased and remained at a low level. For the second child, when the illumination changes were eliminated, switching remained relatively high suggesting that the visual consequence was not a reinforcer. When the clicking sound was removed, switching systematically decreased. This study demonstrated that intervention procedures using extinction for compulsive behavior could only be successful when the procedure used matches the consequence maintaining the compulsive behavior in baseline.

Impulse Control Disorder

Pyromania is often conceived of as an example of an inability to control irresistible impulses to set fires. Kolko, (1983) treated pyromania in a 6-year-old boy with ID. A functional analysis confirmed no apparent antecedents or consequences consistently associated with incidents of fire-setting. It was therefore assumed that automatic sensory reinforcement as well as the possibility that attention from his mother were maintaining the behavior. A multi-component intervention was developed. It consisted of education concerning the characteristics and dangers of fire-setting and reinforcement of alternative activities using tokens and over-correction. Over-correction is a procedure that requires the person to engage in effortful and extensive correction of environmental damage or extensive practice of a correct response many times. Prior to the start of the intervention, the client set four unsanctioned fires. After intervention, no unsanctioned fires were set for 23 weeks. The results were maintained for an additional 15 months.

Attention-Deficit Disorder

Finch, Wilkinson, Nelson, & Montgomery, (1975) assessed the effectiveness of training boys, who were emotionally disturbed and who engaged in impulsive behavior, to practice verbal self-instructions and to wait before responding to tasks. Subjects who were taught to use self-instructions increased their time to respond to tasks and made fewer errors than those in two comparison groups. In a similar study, Bell, Mundy, & Quay, (1983) modified the impulsive responding of 24 boys with severe ID. One group of boys was taught to use five steps to solve a variety of cognitive tasks by modeling. Pennies were given as reinforcement, initially for verbalizing the rules and for correct responses, then ultimately for correct responding only. Results showed that the group had less impulsive responding than when compared to a group of controls. Locher, (1985) used a haptic (active touch) training protocol to modify impulse control in 12 children with communication handicaps as well as neurological impairment. The children were encouraged to use more efficient encoding strategies when solving tasks by direct instruction, modeling, scanning, and search strategies as well as positive verbal reinforcement. After two testing sessions of 30 minutes per child, the children, as a group, improved their encoding strategy and performance on a haptic discrimination task after treatment.

Johnson, Handen, Lubetsky, & Sacco, (1994) used a controlled experiment to compare psychotropic medications and behavioral approaches to managing ADHD. They compared methylphenidate (MPH), a drug commonly prescribed to control impulsive behavior in individuals with ADHD, also commonly referred to as Ritalin, and two behavioral interventions on classroom behavior in three children diagnosed with ADHD and ID. Two behavioral interventions were compared. In the first intervention, tokens were earned every two minutes for on-task behavior, with the opportunity to exchange them after 15 minutes. In the second intervention, there was the addition of an accuracy contingency, whereby each task completed at 100% accuracy after 15 minutes, was also reinforced with tangible items. The results showed that, in general, an accuracy contingency with token economy was most effective. For two out of three subjects, higher dosages of MPH were also beneficial for on-task behavior. Thus, a combination of medication and behavior interventions can be beneficial for children with ID and ADHD, but not medication alone.

Phobias

There is a large body of literature on the effectiveness of ABA with phobias in persons with ID. A wide variety of phobias have been successfully treated including fear of dogs, buses, male doctors, dentists, mannequins, riding in automobiles, escalators, heights, stairs, and entering stores. Treatment of phobias begins with an analysis of the stimuli and situations that evoke fearful responses. Interventions include teaching appropriate coping skills such as relaxation and encouraging self-statements, for example, 'This is scary, but I can cope,' as well as reinforcement for gradually approaching fearful situations without fearful behavior.

Matson, (1981) assessed the fear of entering a grocery store by 12 adults with mild to moderate ID using participant modeling. Before going to the store, the therapist asked subjects to walk through the steps of shopping and to orally report which aspects made them anxious. A hierarchy was then developed. In-vivo sessions were conducted where they were taught how to cope with fear and, if successful, were reinforced with verbal praise. All subjects eventually reached high levels of the adaptive performance.

Addictive Behaviors

Many people with severe and profound ID and people who are closely supervised by their families or residential staff are unlikely to abuse alcohol or other substances. However, individuals with mild ID who live independently may be at an increased risk for substance abuse. This may be because of an inability to identify and resist manipulation, the inability to establish independence, and the lack of knowledge of drug effects. Traditional treatment programs such as Alcoholics Anonymous (AA) may not be effective with individuals with ID. AA depends highly on self-direction, verbal communication, and motivation. These are skills that may be significantly impaired among individuals with ID and mental disorders.

In contrast, behavioral skills' training is applicable to a wide range of individuals (Jerrell & Ridgely, 1995). These programs focus on teaching a variety of prevention and coping skills including self-management skills to maintain abstinence, assertiveness training to handle social pressures toward substance use, coping skills, relapse prevention skills, and problem-solving skills.

Individuals with ID may be at risk to abuse cigarettes. Peine, Darvish, Blakelock, Osborne, & Jensen, (1998) reported an intervention for two institutionalized men. Both exhibited disruptive behavior related to the absence or denial of access to tobacco products. An intervention was implemented where they were able to obtain access to cigarettes if they did not engage in disruptive behavior for a specified amount of time. With initial success, alternative rewards were introduced. The reward that was provided was determined by using a "spinner." Thus, the probability of obtaining cigarettes decreased. This procedure, rather than eliminating smoking, greatly reduced the number of cigarettes that each participant smoked while simultaneously reducing the frequency of disruptive behavior.

Aggression

Aggressive behavior is often inadvertently maintained by the social reaction of others. O'Reilly, Lancioni, & Taylor, (1999) conducted a functional analysis of aggression in a 10-year-old boy with ID. The results of the analysis suggested that his aggression was maintained by attention from others. Based on this hypothesis, they compared two treatments, 1) time-out from attention contingent on the occurrence of aggression and 2) the delivery of noncontingent attention (i.e., the delivery of attention regardless of whether aggression occurred). Both were considered potentially effective treatments in that time-out from attention would make aggression ineffective at obtaining attention from others, whereas noncontingent delivery of attention might reduce the motivational aspects of attention to engage in aggression. O'Reilly et al., (1999) found that noncontingent attention was more effective than time-out. First, the schedule of initial frequent delivery of attention could be gradually faded to relatively infrequent attention. Second, the procedure was easier and more likely to be followed through by the child's parents.

Self-Injurious Behavior

It has long been understood that SIB may be established and maintained by the social behavior of others. Replacing SIB with prosocial behavior is therefore a common goal among clinicians. Inconsistent findings on the efficacy of various procedures, however, have led to a focus on the assessment process prior to intervention as a critical part of developing effective treatments.

The development of methods to identify the functions of SIB led to the development of interventions that can be matched to those functions in each individual. After determining the function, clinicians can identify and teach an alternate response (i.e., FCT), which has the same function as that identified by the functional analysis (Carr & Durand, 1985). Carr et al., (1985) assessed problem behavior, such as self-injury and tantrum behavior, in four children with ID. Following the assessment, the children were taught two responses: "Am I doing good work?" and "I don't understand." The children were first taught to imitate an adult who modeled the responses. This established the children's vocal ability to perform these responses. After the children consistently imitated the responses correctly, they were taught to imitate each response in the correct context. For example, after the child gave an incorrect response to a difficult task, the instructor modeled the response, "I don't understand." Correct imitation of the modeled response was followed by assistance in the task from the teacher. For the response, "Am I doing good work?" the instructor modeled the response for the child after the child had been working on an easy task for 30 seconds without attention from the instructor. Praise statements and physical contact from the teacher were provided following correct imitation of the modeled response. Finally, the modeled responses provided by the instructor were faded by decreasing both the amount and volume of the modeled response. As a result, the children were taught to say, "I don't understand" and "Am I doing good work?" independently in the appropriate and relevant contexts.

Using the same procedures, the children were also taught to provide each response to the "opposite" or irrelevant context. That is, the children were taught to ask, "I don't understand," after they had been working on an easy task and to say, "Am I doing good work?" after giving an incorrect response to a difficult task. The consequences for each of these statements were the same as mentioned above. The purpose of this training was to determine the effect of providing attention in the context of difficult tasks, and the effect of providing assistance in the context of low attention. For example, when presented with a difficult task and the child asked, "Am I doing good work?" the instructor provided attention, but did not provide assistance.

The results showed that when problem behavior was maintained by attention from others, the response, "Am I doing good work?" but not the response "I don't understand" was effective at decreasing problem behavior. Similarly, when problem behavior was maintained by escape-avoidance, the response, "I don't understand" was effective because it resulted in assistance from the instructor. When the contexts were reversed, however, problem behavior occurred at higher rates. These results demonstrate that teaching a functionally equivalent communicative response was effective at decreasing problem behavior.

SUMMARY

ABA involves the systematic investigation of the effect of observable environmental events on the behavior of individuals. The results of these investigations are then used to develop the intervention procedures that are least restrictive to the individual as well as most likely to be effective. ABA uses a variety of methods to collect assessment data, however, direct observation is the predominant method. The main objectives of these data are to understand the relation between the environment and behavior and to develop individually tailored intervention plans to teach more appropriate ways of behaving. While the principles of ABA were identified in studies of animal behavior, the applicability to education and treatment of individuals with mental disorders were clearly indicated. Difficult behaviors that were resistant to other forms of treatment were now treatable by environmental manipulation.

Interventions based on ABA have been used to address a wide range of behaviors exhibited by individuals with mental disorders and ID. Sections in this chapter have described behaviors that are characteristic of various mental disorders and treatments from a behavior analytic perspective. Such studies have identified the critical components for addressing problem behaviors. These include an assessment/analysis of the environmental variables that serve to maintain the target behavior (i.e., the function of the behavior), the development of an intervention that addresses that function directly, the development of an intervention that increases the individual's skill repertoire to the extent that an appropriate behavior replaces the inappropriate behavior, and consideration of the replacement behavior to the extent that it is likely to be maintained by the natural environment (i.e., in the absence of ongoing treatment procedures).

Future research can extend our current knowledge of ABA and its applicability to clients with ID and mental disorders by using functional analysis methodologies and applying the rigorous standards of evaluation more prevalent in research with aggression and SIB to a wider range of diagnoses.

REFERENCES

American Psychiatric Association (2000). *Diagnostic and Statistical Manual of Mental Disorders* (Rev. 4th ed.) Washington, DC: American Psychiatric Association.

Ayllon, T. & Michael, J. (1959). The psychiatric nurse as a behavioral engineer. *Journal of the Experimental Analysis of Behavior, 2*, 323-334.

Baer, D. M., Wolf, M. M., & Risley, T. R. (1968). Some current dimensions of applied behavior analysis. *Journal of Applied Behavior Analysis, 1*, 91 - 97.

Bell, C. R., Mundy, P., & Quay, H. C. (1983). Modifying impulsive responding in conduct-disordered institutionalized boys. *Psychological Reports, 52*, 307-310.

Carr, E. G. & Durand, V. M. (1985). Reducing behavior problems through functional communication training. *Journal of Applied Behavior Analysis, 18*, 111-126.

Didden, R., Duker, P. C., & Korzilius, H. (1997). Meta-analytic study on treatment effectiveness for problem behaviors with individuals who have mental retardation. *American Journal of Mental Retardation, 30*, 387- 399.

Durand, V. M. & Crimmins, D. B. (1987). Assessment and treatment of psychotic speech in an autistic child. *Journal of Autism and Developmental Disorders, 17*, 17-28.

Expert Consensus Panel (2000). Expert Consensus Guideline Series: Treatment of psychiatric and behavioral problems in mental retardation. *American Journal on Mental Retardation, 105*, 159 - 226.

Finch, A. J., Wilkinson, M. D., Nelson III, W. M., & Montgomery, L. E. (1975). Modification of an impulsive cognitive tempo in emotionally disturbed boys. *Journal of Abnormal Child Psychology, 3*, 49-52.

Fuller, P. R. (1949). Operant conditioning of a human vegetative organism. *American Journal of Psychology, 62*, 587-590.

Greenspoon, J. (1955). The reinforcing effect of two spoken words on the frequency of members of two verbal responses. *American Journal of Psychology, 68*, 409-416.

Haughton, E. & Ayllon, T. (1998). The queen's scepter. In P. Chance (Ed.), *First course in applied behavior analysis* (pp. 90-92). Pacific Grove, CA: Brooks/Cole Publishing Company. (Reprinted from Haughton, E. & Ayllon, T. (1965). Production and elimination of symptomatic behavior. In L. P. Ullman & L. Krasner (Eds.) *Case studies in behavior modification*. New York: Holt, Rinehart, and Winston).

Jerrell, J. M. & Ridgely, S. (1995). Comparative effectiveness of three approaches to serving people with severe mental illness and substance abuse disorders. *Journal of Nervous and Mental Disease, 183*, 566-576.

Johnson, C. R., Handen, B. L., Lubetsky, M. J., & Sacco, K. A. (1994). Efficacy of methylphenidate and behavioral intervention on classroom behavior in children with ADHD and mental retardation. *Behavior Modification, 18*, 470-487.

Kolko, D. J. (1983). Multicomponent parental treatment of fire-setting in a six-year-old boy. *Journal of Behavior Therapy and Experimental Psychiatry, 14,* 349-353.

Lindsay, W. R., Howells, L., & Pitcaithly, D. (1993). Cognitive therapy for depression with individuals with intellectual disabilities. *British Journal of Medical Psychology, 66,* 135-141.

Locher, P. J. (1985). Use of haptic training to modify impulse and attention control deficits of learning disabled children. *Journal of Learning Disabilities, 18,* 89-93.

Matson, J. L. (1981). A controlled outcome study of phobias in mentally retarded adults. *Behavior Research and Therapy, 19,* 101-107.

Matson, J. L. (1982). The treatment of behavioral characteristics of depression in the mentally retarded. *Behavior Therapy, 13,* 209-218.

Matson J. L., Baglio, C. S., Smiroldo, B. B., Hamilton, M., Packlowskyi, T., Williams, D., et al. (1996). Characteristics of autism as assessed by the Diagnostic Assessment for the Severely Handicapped-II (DASH-II). *Research In Developmental Disabilities, 17,* 135-143.

New York State Department of Health (1999). *Clinical practice guideline: Quick reference guide for parents and professionals: Autism / pervasive developmental disorders: Assessment and intervention for young children (age 0 - 3 years).* Albany, NY: New York State Department of Health Publications.

O'Neill, R. E., Horner, R. H., Albin, R. W., Sprague, J. R., Storey, K., & Newton, J. S. (1997). *Functional assessment and program development for problem behavior. A practical handbook.* Pacific Grove, CA: Brooks/Cole Publishing Company.

O'Reilly, M., Lancioni, G., & Taylor I. (1999). An empirical analysis of two forms of extinction to treat aggression. *Research in Developmental Disabilities, 20,* 315-325.

Peine, H. A., Darvish, R., Blakelock, H., Osborne, J. G., & Jensen, W. R. (1998). Non-aversive reduction of cigarette smoking in two adult men in a residential setting. *Journal of Behavior Therapy and Experimental Psychiatry, 29,* 55-65.

Rincover, A., Newsom, C. D., & Carr, E. G. (1979). Using sensory extinction procedures in the treatment of compulsive-like behavior of developmentally disabled children. *Journal of Consulting and Clinical Psychology, 47,* 695-701.

Schaefer, H. H. (1970). Self-injurious behavior: Shaping "head-banging" in monkeys. *Journal of Applied Behavior Analysis, 3,* 111-116.

Sarfino, E. P. (2001). *Behavior modification* (2nd ed.). London: Mayfield.

Skinner, B. F. (1938/1999). *The Behavior of Organisms.* Morganton, WV: The Skinner Foundation.

Singh, N. N., Aman, M. G., & Turbott, S. H. (1985). Reliability of the aberrant behavior checklist and the effect of variations in instructions. *American Journal of Mental Deficiency, 92,* 237-240.

Sturmey, P. (1995). Suicidal threats and behavior in a person with developmental disabilities: Effective psychiatric monitoring based on functional assessment. *Behavioral Interventions: Theory and Practice in Residential and Community-Based Clinical Programs, 9,* 235-245.

Sturmey, P., (1996). *Functional Analysis in Clinical Psychology.* London: Wiley.

U. S. Surgeon General (2000). *Mental health: A report of the Surgeon General.* Washington, DC: U. S. Department of Health.

Touchette, P. A., MacDonald, R. F., & Langer, S. N. (1985). A scatterplot for identifying stimulus control of problem behavior. *Journal of Applied Behavior Analysis, 18,* 343-351.

Wacker, D. P., Berg, W. K., Harding, J. W., Derby, K. M., Asmus, J. M., & Healy, A. (1998). Evaluation and long-term treatment of aberrant behavior displayed by young children with disabilities. *Journal of Developmental and Behavioral Pediatrics, 19,* 260-266.

9

Psychotropic Medication

Nancy N. Cain and Anthony Villani

INTRODUCTION

This chapter will provide an overview of medications currently being used to treat individuals with ID and mental or behavioral disorders. At the end, the reader should be familiar with the major classes of medications and special considerations to keep in mind when drugs are used in this population.

Nearly half of all adults with ID are prescribed antipsychotics (formerly called neuroleptics); in people who are institutionalized, this proportion rises to 75%. Psychoactive drugs influence (both positively and negatively) the effectiveness of non-medical treatments such as behavioral modification, special education, or psychotherapy. Medication is just one part of optimum treatment of mental disorders, which should be multimodal and interdisciplinary. Medication should not be used as a substitute for other treatments.

It is important for caregivers to be familiar with the types of medications commonly prescribed as well as their indications and serious side effects. As most individuals now live outside of institutions, where there was quick access to medical personnel, caregivers must now be able to identify the signs of occurring side effects. These caregivers may also be the very people advocating for or against the use of medication, and they should have some understanding of what the medications can and cannot do.

GENERAL PRINCIPLES IN MEDICATION TREATMENT

Assessment and Diagnosis

A complete diagnostic and functional assessment is needed before starting medication. The diagnostic assessment should include:

- A detailed description of the present problems (symptoms);
- All current medications and doses, whether for medical disorders or mental disorders;
- A good mental status examination;
- A complete developmental history including information about pregnancy and delivery, applicable;
- A comprehensive past psychiatric history;
- A listing of previously used medications with a listing, whenever possible, of the benefits, failures, and any adverse reactions of these medications;

- A complete medical history (past and present), and
- A family history of any mental disorders and successful treatments.

It takes time to carefully gather all of the information and understand the symptom presentation in individuals with ID (see Chapter 2). Any possible physical illness, including the presence of pain symptoms, should be investigated and treated. Usually this would be referred to the primary healthcare provider before starting or changing a psychotropic-medication. Ongoing collaboration with all clinicians and caregivers should be established as early as possible.

The Disorder Determines the Medication Used

It is preferable to prescribe medication only after diagnosing a specific mental disorder. A large body of literature based on individuals without ID supports the use of specific medication for groupings of symptoms that clearly meet diagnostic criteria for designated mental disorders. (See Chapters 3 & 4 for discussion of criteria for mental disorders.) Medications for these disorders are usually prescribed in the same way that they are prescribed for individuals without ID. Monitoring may require more help from caregivers. (See below under Importance of Good Data and Methods for Assessing Drug Effectiveness). Sometimes one medication from a class (see Tables 9.2 through 9.7) is not effective. Another one should then be tried, as each medication in a class is slightly different chemically, and individuals respond differently. It may even take a number of trials with medications from a given class before a beneficial effect occurs. Though this can be frustrating, it is both important not to leave someone on a medication that is not effective and to continue to find the best treatment possible. If these trials are unsuccessful, reassess the diagnosis. At times there is a need for several medications in combination, such as an antidepressant, an antipsychotic, and a mood stabilizer for bipolar disorder, before significant improvement is seen.

Aggressive behavior is most responsive to medication when the behavior is associated with a mental disorder that is being treated appropriately. In such cases the aggression is stemming from the disordered thoughts or feelings and should diminish as the disorder is alleviated. Improper treatment of mental disorders often leads to interventions that worsen aggression or side effects.

In autism and other PDD, no drug treatments have been found to effectively treat the core symptoms of the disease. Medications may be useful, however, for a concomitant mental disorder or for severe, disruptive behaviors.

Strategies for Prescribing Medications

Several principles govern the use of psychotropic medications in individuals with ID:
- Though the same doses are generally needed as in the non-ID population, some individuals may not respond as predicted. They may need higher doses, much lower doses, or not respond at all (possibly because the diagnosis is wrong);
- Time is needed to find the most effective medication, and one should not stop after the first few attempts;
- Sometimes a combination of medications will be more effective than any one medication alone;

- "Start low, go slow." Use lower initial doses and raise doses slowly to both decrease side effects and allow earlier recognition of when they occur;
- Dose reductions should also be gradual to allow time for the body to adjust and prevent withdrawal or rebound side effects;
- Monitor and evaluate the need for a given medication for possible dose reduction or elimination of medications at regular intervals. "Drug holidays," simply to reduce the life-time dose of medication received, can be harmful and may make it difficult to return to the level of functioning present before the medication was stopped;
- Avoid frequent drug and dose changes unless necessary to avoid side effects, and
- Use evidence-based principles whenever possible.

Importance of Good Data

Without an organized system for tracking behavior or symptoms, it is difficult to assess the effects of psychotropic medications. When caregivers rely on memory they are often influenced by the most recent events. Without recorded data over time, a significant decrease in the behaviors may not be recognized if the behaviors are still occurring, although at a lower level. This could lead to a change to a different medication rather than an increase to attain further efficacy. As well, different caregivers remember events differently. It is important for multidisciplinary teams to develop and implement tools to measure baseline behaviors and monitor both the positive and negative effects of medication in a consistent way (Sovner & Hurley, 1987). There are a variety of tools, described below, that can be helpful. It is important to track symptoms that the medication is expected to eliminate as well as potential side effects.

METHODS FOR ASSESSING DRUG EFFECTIVENESS

Global Impressions Scales

These scales rate behavior change in terms of the rater's subjective impressions of the client. They are useful as general screens to detect drug effects but can be subject to bias in the rater's impressions. Examples include the Clinical Global Impression Scale (CGI), Overt Aggression Scale (OAS), and Conner's Scale for ADHD. These scales are available in most textbooks or online.

Direct Behavioral Observations

Here, to be objective and clear and to eliminate as much rater bias as possible, target behaviors are described precisely and documented each time they occur. Observational data is then collected and organized, often through graphing. Change in frequency of the target behaviors from baseline (measured before the medication is started) is then tracked. Education of all caregivers must precede the implementation of this type of assessment. An example of this would be agitation. The staff and treating clinician would need to agree upon what constituted agitation. For one individual it might be pacing for more than 10 minutes; for another it might include yelling and screaming without responding to redirection. Verbal threats might be included but generally should be recorded as a separate item. They may not occur as often or could mean something else such as being more upset than usual or having hallucinations

Assessing Side Effects

Medications should be evaluated regularly to determine if side effects are both present and compromising functional status. Reviews should occur at least every 6 to 12 months for stable individuals but should occur more frequently (e.g., weekly to monthly) after new medications are begun or doses changed (Reiss & Aman, Eds., 1998). Standardized assessment instruments, scales, or checklists such as the CGI could be useful in monitoring adverse drug effects (Reiss et al., 1998).

In general, particular attention should be given to observed changes in:
- Activities of daily living such as locomotion, bathing, or dressing;
- Cognition or thinking, especially memory and orientation;
- Communication (verbal and nonverbal);
- Continence of bladder and bowel, or
- Interest in favorite activities and motivation.

There are a number of rating scales that are widely available tools designed to focus on a particular area of functioning, behavior, or side effect. They include tools like the Overt Aggression Scale (OAS) (Yudofsky, Silver, Jackson, Endicott, & Williams, 1986) to measure the frequency and intensity of aggression; the Abnormal Involuntary Movement Scale (AIMS) (Munetz & Benjamin, 1988) to assess for extra pyramidal side effects, and the Yale–Brown Obsessive Compulsive Scale (Y-BOCS) (Goodman et al., 1989) for obsessions and compulsions.

Caregivers can do some of the evaluations such as the direct-behavioral data collection; clinicians should do the AIMS, and the Y-BOCS is administered by the clinician by asking questions of the client or caregiver(s).

Use of Multiple Medications and Drug-Drug Interactions

As described previously, most people with ID and a mental disorder are on multiple medications. Often this is justified and necessary to treat the multiple problems of a particular client. However, it is important not to engage in *polypharmacy* (use of more than one medication from the same class), unless the benefits are well documented. Consequences of polypharmacy include the potential for a much higher incidence of side effects, increased drug costs, and worsening of cognitive difficulties.

Even when multiple medications are justified, their interactions with each other in the individual client must be considered. The possibility of significant drug-drug interactions increases exponentially as more medications are added to a client's treatment. Drugs may interact in such a way as to interfere with their effectiveness and diminish treatment or lead to unexpected toxicity. For example, a common drug that increases the liver's rate of metabolism such as Tegretol (carbamazepine) may speed up the liver's breakdown of other medications. This can lead to a decrease in the effect of the other medication and a potential increase in symptoms. A drug such as a selective serotonin reuptake inhibitor (SSRI) can block a liver enzyme and decrease the liver's rate of metabolism or breakdown of other medications. Adding such a drug to a client's regimen may effectively "increase" the dose of pre-existing medications and lead to toxic side effects. Another such example is the combination of a monoamine oxidase inhibitor (MAOI) and a tricyclic, which can lead to a life-threatening elevation of the individual's blood pressure. A drug that increases the kidney's rate of excretion may decrease the duration of another medication in a client's system, leading to what appears to be the loss of its effectiveness. On the other hand, the simple addition of an antibiotic like penicillin or a pain reliever such as ibuprofen may interfere with the kidney's clearance of lithium, leading to lithium toxicity.

As the total number of a client's medications increases (including non-psychotropic medications), drug interactions become harder to predict. Caregivers should regularly review medication lists and consider potential interactions. References, including books like the *Physicians' Desk Reference* (PDR), the *Nurse's Prescribing Handbook*, or software like the *Adverse Drug Interactions Program* should be widely available to check for common drug-drug interactions. The pharmacist that supplies the medication is also a good resource. Any or all of these references and resources should be consulted whenever a new medication is prescribed, when a previously effective medication seems to lose its potency, when a prescribed medication does not work as predicted, or when an old medication is stopped.

Strategies To Reduce Medication Use

A general goal for treatment with psychotropic medications is to find the lowest maintenance dose(s) possible that still produce(s) the intended effect. Reduction strategies should include:

- Review of medication lists regularly to consider the necessity of the medication;
- Reassess of medications any time diagnoses are changed or life changes occur;
- Objectively identify target behaviors and symptoms with careful monitoring during a drug taper;
- Return to the prior dose if symptoms recur, BEFORE they become severe; if there is too much deterioration in an individual's behavior and/or functioning, it may be difficult to achieve as effective a response as before the taper began;
- Document side effects and any changes that occur;
- Observe for any withdrawal symptoms such as nausea, anxiety, or agitation that may occur, and
- Discontinue medications gradually to allow the body to readjust.

When there is clear documentation that an individual decompensates without a particular medication, there should be no further attempts to stop the medication as the disorder itself may cause more adverse effects. A risk benefit analysis should be done regularly to determine whether the potential side effects or the benefit of the symptom relief is greater.

Strategies for Changing Medication
Key Points:
- **Avoid making multiple medication changes at the same time.**
  Medication changes are a common occurrence in modern medicine as drugs initially chosen may not lead to full remission of symptoms; new ones become available, or individuals develop side effects. Whether altering the dose of an existing medication, adding a new drug, or discontinuing medication:

- **Avoid making multiple changes simultaneously, whenever possible.**
  If two or more drug changes are made at the same time, benefits or side effects that arise often cannot be clearly attributed to a particular medication.
- **Carefully plan and monitor overlap or crossover periods.**
  Sometimes a new medication is substituted for another that targets the same symptoms. For example, a typical antipsychotic may be changed to a newer atypical antipsychotic. The new agent is usually added to the old agent for an *overlap* period, and then the older agent is gradually discontinued. This strategy avoids the possibility that the client's stability is jeopardized during the change. Also, using an overlap period clarifies whether a change is due to the discontinuation of the first drug or the start of the second.
- **Make the length of the overlap period as short as possible to limit the additive effects of multiple medications but long enough to prevent relapse.**

USE OF MEDICATIONS IN VULNERABLE POPULATIONS

Informed Consent

The capacity of a person with ID and a mental disorder to understand and give consent to treatment should be assessed on a case-by-case basis. Every use of medication should follow a discussion of benefits, risks, and side effects with the client, parent, or guardian. Ethical issues in treatment are discussed in greater detail in Chapter 11.

Use of Medications for Restraint

Psychotropic medications continue to be used in practice as an alternative to physical restraint in situations where a client's behavior poses a risk to himself/herself or others. To avoid abuses, especially in chronically understaffed residential settings for those with ID and mental disorders, caregivers must familiarize themselves with the Mental Health policy of their particular state, province, or region. In general, restraints, whether physical or chemical, are justified only when the following two criteria are met (Simon, 1998):

- They are needed to prevent clear, imminent harm to the client or others, or, rarely, at the client's voluntary reasonable request, and
- Restraints are "the least restrictive alternative," i.e., other, less invasive steps have been tried unsuccessfully, and alternatives to restraint have been exhausted.

Children

There is much less information available on the safety and effectiveness of drugs in children. Children are not "little adults," they have differences in how they absorb, distribute, and metabolize medication. This is related in part to their smaller body mass, and thus the milligrams of medication per kilograms of weight become important in avoiding a toxic dose. As children grow rapidly, dosing of medication is often given on a per kilogram basis. At times, a medication that seems to lose effectiveness may be a result of a child outgrowing his daily dose. Children should be weighed regularly (e.g., every six months) and doses adjusted for weight gain and increased body mass.

Older and Aging Adults

Many of the physical changes associated with aging affect how medications work in the elderly. Age-related changes in the kidney and liver can lead to limited kidney or liver function. This means that medications are often metabolized more slowly and not cleared from the body as quickly as in younger adults. As a result, lower doses are generally required.

Often geriatric practitioners start at a fraction of the usual FDA-approved starting dose and make changes over the course of weeks or months, not days. The mantra "start low, go slow" is a good rule of thumb for dosing medication in these clients. Before adding medication in an older client, the caregiver should be familiar with any underlying medical problems and other medications that the individual is taking. Older adults are often less able to tolerate side effects such as blurred vision, dry mouth, and constipation. Drugs may significantly alter cognition or cause light headache and lead to a greater risk of falling. Individuals should be watched closely for such problems, and medications should be altered accordingly.

Pregnancy

Many of the psychotropic medications can lead to birth defects if taken during pregnancy. Depakote, a commonly used mood stabilizer, has been shown to increase the risk of spinal bifida in infants whose mothers took the drug during the first trimester. Table 9.1 shows the FDA's classification of pregnancy risk of all prescription drugs using a letter system A, B, C, D, and X. Current or suspected pregnancy in a client should prompt a review of the client's current medications to look for any possible risks.

TABLE 9.1
FDA Rating of Drug Safety in Pregnancy*

Category	Definition	Drug Example
A	No fetal risks in controlled human studies	Iron
B	No fetal risk in animal studies but no adequate human studies	Acetaminophen
C	Adverse fetal effects in animals and no human data available	Aspirin, Haloperidol
D	Human fetal risk seen (may be used in life-threatening situation)	Lithium, Ethanol
X	Proved fetal risk in humans (no indication for use, even in life-threatening situations)	Valproic acid, Thalidomide

* Adapted from FDA, 2001

DRUG CLASSES

The following is a brief summary of most of the classes of medications used to treat mental disorders. In each section, many of the more common or life-threatening side effects are mentioned. However, this is not an all-inclusive listing. Resources such as the information sheets that pharmacies include with medications or the *Physicians' Desk Reference* (PDR) should be consulted.

Antipsychotics

This class of medications is divided into two groups: the typical and the atypical (see below). These drugs are commonly used to:
- Reduce hallucinations, paranoia, and delusional thoughts associated with disorders like schizophrenia and bipolar disorder;
- Decrease aggression stemming from mental disorders;
- Control anger or aggression acutely by slowing down the motor system;
- Treat tics, stereotyped motor behaviors, Tourette's disorder;
- Treat anxiety and agitation not responsive to other anti-anxiety medications.

Typical Antipsychotics

Table 9.2 shows the most common typical antipsychotic medications. These pharmaceuticals have been used for decades. The most recognized example is haloperidol. Haloperidol and fluphenazine have depot preparations that are long-acting injections that can be administered every 1 to 4 weeks. They can be very useful when medication compliance cannot be assured, or in cases where clients chronically refuse to take oral medication.

TABLE 9.2
Typical Antipsychotics

Generic	Trade Name (US)	Usual Dosage Range
Fluphenazine	Prolixin, Permitil	0.05 mg. – 10 mg.
Haloperidol	Haldol	2 mg. – 20 mg.
Thiothixene	Navane	10 mg. – 60 mg.
Trifluperizine	Stelazine	10 mg. – 40 mg.
Pimozide	Orap	2 mg. – 20 mg.
Molindone	Moban	50 mg. – 225 mg.
Perphenazine	Trilafon	12 mg. – 64 mg.
Loxapine	Loxitane	50 mg. – 250 mg.
Mesoridazine	Serentil	150 mg. – 400 mg.
Chlorpromazine	Thorazine	100 mg. – 1000 mg.
Thioridazine	Mellaril	25 mg. – 800 mg.

Atypical Antipsychotics

Table 9.3 shows common atypical antipsychotic medications. These newer medications are called "atypical" because they work differently and have somewhat different side effects than the older "typical" antipsychotics. One significant difference is that the newer agents not only treat hallucinations and aggression, but they also may help with the negative symptoms of psychotic illness such as social withdrawal, blunted affect, and lack of motivation. They are significantly more expensive than the typical antipsychotics, but thought to be less likely to cause the side effects of tardive dyskinesia (TD): slow, writhing or tic-like involuntary movements, usually beginning in the tongue or facial muscles (see below). They may also be tolerated better and thus lead to less non-compliance.

TABLE 9.3
Atypical Antipsychotics*

Generic	Trade Name (US)	Usual Dosage Range
Clozapine	Clozaril	100 mg. – 500 mg.
Olanzapine	Zyprexa	2.5 mg. – 40 mg.
Quetiapine	Seroquel	25 mg. – 1000 mg.
Risperidone	Risperdal	0.25 mg. – 16 mg.
Ziprasidone	Geodon	20 mg. – 160 mg.
Aripiprazole	Abilify	10 mg. – 45 mg.

* Dosage maximums are still being established. In some, difficult-to-treat individuals, higher doses may be used when there is literature to support it.

Side Effects Of Antipsychotic Medications

Most side effects of antipsychotic medications are the same whether typical or atypical antipsychotics. The occurrence frequency of each of the side effects listed below varies for each drug and often influences the one chosen for a particular individual. It is currently felt that the atypical antipsychotic medications will not cause tardive dyskinesia, but this conclusion may change with the findings that higher doses are needed for the most difficult-to-treat individuals.

Some side effects of antipsychotics occur commonly (i.e., in many people taking the medication), while others are only moderately common.

Common side effects include:

- Sedation (which often decreases after the first two weeks);
- Weight gain;
- Dry mouth and constipation;
- Amenorrhea, the absence of menstruation;
- Decreased libido, and
- Low blood pressure (especially when moving from lying to sitting or sitting to standing).

Moderately common side effects include:

- Extrapyramidal symptoms (EPS): Acute side effects such as muscle spasms, called *dystonias*, or pacing and restlessness, called *akathisia*. Often these side effects will

mimic the symptoms of Parkinson's disease, including tremor, stooped posture, shuffling gait, and slowness in initiating movements;
- Increased seizure activity: Antipsychotics should be used cautiously in individuals with seizure disorders as they can lower the seizure threshold and cause more seizures. Often collaborative work with a neurologist can ensure the effective control of both the seizures and the psychotic disorder. Rarely, a seizure disorder may occur in someone who has never had a seizure;
- Moderate to severe weight gain, and
- Increased glucose and lipid levels (Wirshing et al., 2002).

Potentially life-threatening side effects include:
- Decreased red or white blood cells: This most often occurs with Clozapine, which is known to dangerously lower the white blood cell counts and needs monitoring by blood tests every 1 to 2 weeks. This occurs less often with other antipsychotic medications but should be assessed every 6 to 12 months;
- Tardive Dyskinesia: Serious long-term effects such as uncontrollable movements of the jaw, tongue, lips, or extremities. It may affect the muscles of swallowing and respiration. It generally occurs after months or years of treatment with typical antipsychotics. It may not become evident until the medication is stopped. The risk increases the longer the antipsychotics are used and the higher the lifetime dose. Thus, the benefit of the medication (relief from impairment and distress from the disorder) and the risks (disability caused by the medication) must be reviewed regularly. The lowest dose possible should be used for maintenance;
- Increased QTc interval: This is a measure on the electrocardiogram of the cardiac conduction. If significantly increased it can lead to a life-threatening arrhythmia. Proper prescribing of antipsychotic drugs with this side effect, especially ziprasidone and thioridazine, should follow a review of a client's medical history and may require an initial electrocardiogram (ECG) as well as a follow-up one in 6 months; or
- Neuroleptic malignant syndrome (NMS) (Guze & Baxter, 1985): NMS consists of high fever, muscle rigidity and confusion. NMS is a medical emergency that must be treated at a hospital. Any suspicion of these side effects should be reported immediately, since early detection and treatment can prevent potentially life-threatening outcomes.

Mood Stabilizers

These medications are used in clients with bipolar disorder. Many of these medications were originally used in treating epilepsy and later found to be useful for treating irritability, aggression, and mood swings when part of a bipolar disorder. Table 9.4 gives the most common mood stabilizers.

Clients with underlying brain damage are more likely to have rapid cycling of mood symptoms, or "mixed" affective states, where some symptoms of both mania and depression are present at the same time (Santosh & Baird, 1999). Mood stabilizers are the mainstay of treatment for these symptoms.

TABLE 9.4
Common Mood Stabilizers

Generic	Trade Name (US)	Usual Dosage Range
Lithium	Eskalith, Lithobid	600 mg. – 1800 mg.
Valproic Acid	Depakote	250 mg. – 3000 mg.
Carbamazepine	Tegretol, Carbitrol	600 mg. – 1800 mg.
Lamotrigine	Lamictal	100 mg. – 500 mg.
Oxcarbazepine	Trileptal	600 mg. – 2400 mg.
Topiramate	Topamax	100 mg. – 400 mg.

Careful monitoring of these medications is required. Initially, several tests must be conducted to make certain that side effects will not worsen an existing condition and put the client's health at risk. These medications take time to reach the appropriate dose, as too little of the drug will often fail to treat behaviors while too much can be toxic to the client. Prescribers aim to maintain the concentration of the mood stabilizer in a narrow range. Blood level monitoring is available for lithium, carbamazepine, and valproic acid. These blood tests are frequently done initially and as often as every 3 to 6 months for maintenance treatment. The other mood stabilizers are monitored clinically for improvement or side effects.

Side Effects For Lithium:
- Often causes tremors, weight gain, increased thirst, and the need to urinate, and
- Over time, chronic lithium therapy can be toxic to the thyroid gland and kidney, causing hypo or hyperthyroidism and/or renal impairment. Blood tests to monitor thyroid and kidney functioning must be done yearly in men and every 6 months in women, who are at higher risk of developing changes in these two body systems.

Side Effects for Anticonvulsants:
- Weight gain may occur;
- Cognitive side effects may occur including problems with memory and concentration. These side effects are often more severe initially, with subsequent adaptation over time;
- Lower red blood cells, lower white blood cells, and lower platelets can occur at any time, as can impairment of liver functioning. Blood work is needed frequently initially and then yearly or when clinical symptoms warrant;
- Rashes can occur and are important as they may progress to a life-threatening skin reaction called Stevens-Johnson syndrome. Therefore, any rash should be reported immediately, and
- Most anticonvulsants can interfere with effectiveness of birth control pills and calcium absorption. Calcium supplements can help the latter. Coordination with a gynecologist is important for the former.

As with most medications, the best strategy to limit the extent of side effects is to start with low doses and increase gradually. Often high doses are needed in the acute phase and can be lowered for maintenance treatment.

Antidepressants

These medications are used primarily to treat depression. Table 9.5 depicts the most common antidepressants. Antidepressants should be given for an additional 6 to 12 months after an episode of depression has resolved. Long-term maintenance treatment is recommended when depression is recurrent. The medications require 2 to 6 weeks use to show effectiveness. Since side effects are often worse initially, during this time clients and caregivers need more frequent contact with the therapist, education about the side effects, and reassurance.

Antidepressant medications can trigger manic symptoms in clients with bipolar disorder. It is important to recognize symptoms of mania (irritability, grandiosity, euphoria, and hyperactivity) before and during treatment of clients for depression.

TABLE 9.5
Antidepressants

Generic Name	Trade Name (US)	Usual Dosage Range
TRICYCLICS		
Amityrptiline	Elavil	150 mg – 300 mg
Clomipraine	Anafranil	150 mg – 300 mg
Desipraine	Norpramin	100 mg – 300 mg
Doxepin	Sinaquan	75 mg – 300 mg
Imipriamine	Trofanil	100 mg – 300 mg
Nortriptlyine	Aventyl, Pamelor	75 mg – 300 mg
Protriptyline	Vivactil	15 mg – 60 mg
Trimipramine	Surmontil	50 mg – 200 mg
SSRIs		
Citralopram	Celexa	10 mg – 60 mg
Escitalopram	Lexapro	10 mg. – 20 mg.
Fluoxetine	Prozac	10 mg – 80 mg
Fluvoxamine	Luvox	100 mg – 300 mg
Paroxetine	Paxil	20 mg – 50 mg
Sertraline	Zoloft	50 mg – 200 mg
OTHER ANTIDEPRESSANTS		
Bupropion	Wellbutrin, Wellbutrin SR	150 mg – 300 mg
Mirtazapine	Remeron, RemeronSolTab	30 mg – 45 mg
Nafazodone	Serzone	200 mg – 600 mg
Venlafaxine	Effexor, Effexor XR	75 mg – 225 mg

Tricyclic Antidepressants

These are one of the older types of antidepressants and are still widely used. Pharmacologically they affect different neurotransmitters than the newer medications.

Side Effects include:
- Sedation often occurs, thus they are sometimes given at night to promote sleep;
- Postural hypotension can lead to falls, which limits their use in the elderly;
- Effects similar to anticholinergic drugs (see below) may occur, and
- Overdose can cause life-threatening cardiac arrhythmias. There use can be problematic in those who are suicidal.

Serotonin Specific Reuptake Inhibitors (SSRIs)

The most commonly used antidepressants are called SSRIs. These medications increase the availability of serotonin, a neurotransmitter, in the brain. They are used to treat depression, obsessive-compulsive disorder (OCD), generalized anxiety disorder (GAD), panic disorder, and posttraumatic stress disorder (PTSD). They are relatively safer than other antidepressants, with little potential for life-threatening consequences from regular use or even overdose.

Most common side effects (generally mild):
- Nausea
- Vomiting
- Headache
- Anxiety
- Weight gain

Many of these side effects resolve after 2 to 3 weeks.

Other side effects:
- Decreased libido
- Delayed ejaculation in men and inability to have an orgasm in women
- Serotonin discontinuation syndrome
    - Caused by stopping the medication quickly;
    - Most common symptoms are nausea, anxiety, flu-like symptoms, headache, or dizziness, and
    - Return to taking the medication stops the symptoms.
- Serotonin syndrome
    - Caused by the presence of a toxic amount of serotonin;
    - Is rare and usually occurs as a result of the simultaneous use of two or more medications that increase serotonin levels in the brain, and
    - Examples are an SSRI and dextromethorphan or pseudoephedrine (Lane & Baldwin, 1997), which are found in many over-the-counter cold remedies. (For symptoms of serotonin syndrome see Table 9.6.)

TABLE 9.6	
Serotonin Syndrome Symptoms	
• Shivering • Tremor • Increased Temperature • Sweating	• Muscle Rigidity • Increased Reflexes • Increased Heart Rate (pulse) • Agitation
These may progress to: • Hallucinations* • Seizures* • Confusion* • Coma*	
Medical attention should be sought immediately if any of these four symptoms* occur.	

Other Antidepressants

Bupropion has been effective in the agitated depression that occurs in individuals with bipolar disorder. It is less likely than other antidepressants to cause the switch into mania. It has gained favor as an alternative for the treatment of ADHD as well. Its primary side effects are agitation, decreased appetite, insomnia, and tremor. Seizures may occur with very high doses or in individuals who already have a seizure disorder.

Trazodone is quite sedating and often used as a sleeping aid rather than an antidepressant.

Venlafaxine is often used in cases of severe depression or when the depression is unresponsive to other drugs (Nierenberg, Feighner, Rudolph, Cole, & Sullivan, 1994). Increased blood pressure occurs in some people with higher doses and must be closely monitored initially.

MAOIs (isocarboxazid, phenelzine, and tranylcipromine,) are generally not used in individuals with ID, because the diet must be carefully controlled to prevent a significant increase in blood pressure if foods high in tyramine are eaten. Common side effects of MAOIs include orthostatic hypotension and weight gain.

Anti-Anxiety Drugs (Anxiolytics)

This class contains benzodiazepines and other agents such as those shown in Table 9.7. They are best used in conjunction with therapy to teach coping skills such as relaxation techniques or interpersonal skills. Anxiety symptoms can occur independently or as part of another mental disorder such as depression, obsessive-compulsive disorder, or psychosis. Chronic use of benzodiazepines can lead to dependence, so these medications are best used to control acute anxiety reactions. However, sometimes use of a long-acting benzodiazepine like clonazepam can decrease the amount of antipsychotic medication needed for an individual with bipolar disorder. They may also be the best sleep medication for some individuals. Side effects of benzodiazepines include daytime sedation and motor incoordination. Very rarely they can cause disinhibition, which may cause some individuals to become aggressive.

TABLE 9.7
Anxiolytics

Generic	Trade Name (US)	Usual Oral Dosage Range
Alprazolam	Xanax	0.25 mg. – 4 mg.
Buspirone	Buspar	15 mg. – 45 mg.
Chlordiazepoxide	Librium	15 mg. – 100 mg.
Clonazepam	Klonopin	0.5 mg. – 8 mg.
Clorazepate	Tranxene	15 mg. – 60 mg.
Diazepam	Valium	2.5 mg. – 40 mg.
Hydroxyzine	Vistaril/Atarax	50 mg. – 200 mg.
Lorazepam	Ativan	0.5 mg. – 4 mg.
Oxazepam	Serax	30 mg. – 120 mg.

Drugs Used To Treat Attention Deficit/Hyperactivity Disorder (ADHD)

Drugs are commonly used to treat symptoms of hyperactivity when part of ADHD. Methylphenidate and dexamphetamine are widely prescribed, and since 2000 many newer agents have been introduced, including Focalin, Ritalin LA, Concerta, and Strattera. Clonidine and bupropion, while not stimulants, have also been found to be effective in some cases. Stimulant drugs paradoxically improve attention, focus, and concentration, while reducing fidgeting, pacing, and other hyperactive symptoms. Given their abuse potential, they are controlled substances. Stimulants are common ingredients in over-the-counter appetite suppressants, no-doze drugs used by students and truckers, and over-the-counter cold remedies.

The most common side effects are appetite suppression and insomnia. Psychostimulants also exacerbate tics, seizures, anxiety, and psychotic symptoms and should be used cautiously in clients with these symptoms.

Sleeping Aids/Hypnotics

Sleep disturbances are very common in mental disorders, medical illness, and organic brain damage. Behavioral interventions are a mainstay of treatment. They include calming activities before bedtime, not using the bedroom for other activities, not napping during the day, decreasing the stress in the environment, decreasing the stress in the individual's life, and finding things that are conducive to sleep in the individual such as drinking warm milk, taking a warm bath, or having a calming story read (HCFA, 1996).

A variety of medications have been commonly used, primarily for their "side effects" of sedation. These would include sedating antidepressants such as trazodone, imipramine, and mirtazapine; sedating antihistamines like diphenhydramine and chloral hydrate, and benzodiazepines like clonazepam and lorazepam. These cause a deep sleep without the usual REM cycles that occur during sleep. This makes it difficult to terminate these medications, as individuals often find it difficult to return to the REM phases, which increase initially ("rebound effect") and may lead to increased dreaming or lighter sleep. Attempts have been made to develop more specific sleeping medications. These include zolpidem and zaleplon.

Anticholinergic Drugs

Several classes of psychotropic medications, such as tricyclic antidepressants or atypical antipsychotics, have anticholinergic side effects including dry mouth and sedation. Additionally, drugs with primarily anticholinergic effects, such as trihexylphenidyl and benztropine, are often used in conjunction with antipsychotics to reduce the extrapyramidal side effects (Goff et al., 1991; Sramek, Simpson, Morrison, & Heiser, 1986).

These medications are sedating and should be given at bedtime. They have a distinct set of side effects related to blocking the activity of the parasympathetic nervous system.

They are:
- Constipation,
- Dry mouth and eyes,
- Urinary retention (which can lead to incontinence),
- Dizziness, especially when arising from a bed or chair, and
- Rapid heart rate.

These medications may also lead to cognitive changes including confusion, drowsiness, and memory or concentration problems. Cognitive side effects should be suspected any time that clients have mental status changes soon after anticholinergic drugs are given.

Beta-Blockers

Drugs in this class (examples include propranolol, nadolol, and pindolol) were originally used in medicine to reduce blood pressure and heart rate. Some studies show they are helpful to reduce impulsiveness, stereotypies, aggressive behavior, and self-injury (Ratey et al., 1986). Yet, they are not commonly used, mainly because they can drop blood pressure and heart rate to dangerously low levels in otherwise healthy clients. This especially becomes a problem during exercise, since the usual rise in pulse rate is blunted and leads to inadequate oxygenation. Beta-blockers are known to increase the risk of depression. Any mood changes or vital sign changes should be recorded and reported immediately.

SUMMARY

Psychotropic medications are an important part of the treatment for mental disorders. They can make a significant difference to an individual's quality of life when they are used carefully and thoughtfully. As noted throughout this book, they are more effective after a complete, detailed assessment is conducted and an informed diagnosis made. Once this is done, medication choices are made in the same way as for individuals without ID. However, because many people with ID cannot clearly describe their response to the medication, care must be taken to define and record behavioral information that will reflect their actual response. Responses to new medications must be monitored frequently to determine the appropriate effective dose. If there is no improvement after a reasonable trial, the medication should be stopped and, if necessary, another one tried. The right environment is also important. No medication can overcome the effects of a stressful living or working situation.

REFERENCES

Goff, D. C., Arana, G. W., Greenblatt, D. J., Dupont, R., Ornsteen, M., Harmatz, J., et al. (1991). The effect of benztropine on haloperidol-induced dystonia, clinical efficacy and pharmacokinetics: A prospective double-blind trial. *Journal of Clinical Psychopharmacology, 11*, 106.

Goodman, W. K., Price, L. H., Rasmussen, S. A., Mazure, C., Fleischmann, R. L., Hill, C. L., et al. (1989). The Yale-Brown Obsessive Compulsive Scale, Part I: Development, use, and reliability. *Archives of General Psychiatry, 46*, 1006-1011.

Guze, B. H. & Baxter, L. R. (1985). Current concept: Neuroleptic malignant syndrome. *The New England Journal of Medicine, 313,* 163-166.

Health Care Financing Administration, (1996). *Dealing with insomnia: Report on question 14 and health standards and quality bureau center for long-term care* (pp. 1-14). Baltimore: U.S. Dept. of Health and Human Services.

Lane, R. & Baldwin, D. (1997). Selective serotonin reuptake inhibitor-induced serotonin syndrome: Review. *Journal of Clinical Psychopharmacology, 17,* 208-219.

Munetz, M. R., & Benjamin, S. (1988). How to examine patients using the abnormal involuntary movement scale. *Hospital and community psychiatry, 39*, 1172-1177.

Nierenberg, A. A., Feighner, J. P., Rudolph, R., Cole, J. O., & Sullivan, J. (1994). Venlafaxine for treatment-resistant unipolar depression. *Journal of Clinical Psychopharmacology, 14*, 419.

Sifton, D. W. (Ed.). (2003). *Physicians' Desk Reference* (57th ed.). Montvale, NJ: Thomson.

Ratey, J. J., Mikkelsen, E. J., & Smith, G. B., Upadhyaya, A., Zuckerman, H. S., Martell, D., et al. (1986). Beta-Blockers in the severely and profoundly mentally retarded. *Journal of Clinical Psychopharamacology, 6,* 103-07.

Reiss, S. & Aman, M. G. (Eds.). (1998). *The International Consensus Handbook: Psychotropic medication and developmental disabilities* (p. 61). Columbus, OH: The Ohio State University Nisonger Center.

Santosh, P. & Baird, G. (1999). Psychopharmacotherapy in children and adults with intellectual disability. *The Lancet, 354*, 233-242.

Simon, R. I. (1998). *Concise guide to psychiatry and the law for clinicians* (2nd ed.). Washington, DC: American Psychiatric Press.

Sovner, R., & Hurley, A. D. (1987). Objective behavioral monitoring of psychotropic drug therapy. *Psychiatric Aspects of Intellectually Disability Reviews, 6,* 48-51.

Sramek, J. J., Simpson, G. M., Morrison, R. L., & Heiser, J. F. (1986). Anticholinergic agents for the prophylaxis of neuroleptic-induced dystonic reactions: A prospective study. *Journal of Clinical Psychiatry, 47*, 305.

Wirshing, D. A., Boyd, J. A., Meng, L. R., Ballon, J. S., Marder, S. R., & Wirshing, W. C. (2002). The effects of novel antipsychotics on glucose and lipid levels. *Journal of Clinical Psychiatry, 63*, 856-865.

Yudofsky, S. C., Silver, J. M., Jackson, W., Endicott, J., & Williams, D. (1986). The overt aggression scale for the objective rating of verbal and physical aggression. *American Journal of Psychiatry, 143*, 35-39.

10

Community-Based Mental Health Services

Nick Bouras, Geraldine Holt, and Amy Cowley

INTRODUCTION

This chapter is concerned with the service factors for people with ID, who also have a mental disorder, which may or may not be manifested by behavior problems. People with ID are estimated to be three to four times more likely than those in the general population to experience an emotional, behavioral, or mental disorder (Deb, Matthews, Holt, & Bouras, 2001). The mental health of people with ID has received increasing attention over the last two decades, and there has been a growing consensus to respond more adequately to the needs of those people with a mental disorder and ID. A number of industrialized countries, such as the U.K. and U.S., have been developing and promoting clinical services, specialist training, and research in this field. As a result, specific diagnostic tools have been developed such the Psychiatric Assessment Schedule for Adults with Developmental Disabilities (PAS-ADD) (Moss et al., 1998) which, combined with an increasing knowledge of clinical presentation, has led to an improvement in the assessment and diagnosis of mental disorders in those with ID. The effectiveness of comprehensive therapeutic approaches incorporating behavioral, analytic, and cognitive behavioral component strategies have been demonstrated with a range of behavior and mental disorders, particularly among those with mild or moderate ID (Dosen, 1993; Gardner, Graeber, & Cole, 1996; Gardner & Whalen, 1996).

Organizations such as The European Association for Mental Health in Intellectual Disabilities and The National Association for the Dually Diagnosed (NADD) in the U.S. have been established and have published practice guidelines and training manuals for those with an ID and mental disorders.

POLICY AND PLANNING

The main focus of policy since the 1960s has been the reduction of people with ID living in any kind of institutional care and the rapid development of alternative community services. The implementation of policy for new service developments has been varied in the different parts of the world. In most industrialized countries such as the U.S., U.K., Canada, Australia, and Scandinavia, deinstitutionalization programs have been well advanced. For example, in the U.S., the number of people with ID living in institutional care fell by 46%

between 1976 and 1996 (Jacobson, 1998). Other places, particularly non-industrialized countries, have lacked impetus, and services are not so advanced (Hatton, Emerson, & Kiernan, 1995). Achievements of community care include the development of a wide range of residential settings, respite care, daytime activities, employment opportunities, and mainstream education. Allen & Felce (1999) found that a variety of positive outcomes from the closure of institutions have been demonstrated for those residents concerned. However, there are considerable differences in observed results (Emerson & Hatton, 1995). Positive outcomes include: improved models of social care, enabling clients and their families to be more involved in their own care, and improved integration with the local community—perhaps through attending local churches, participating in adult education classes, and taking up paid work. Mental disorders may be an important factor affecting adaptation to community life, limiting quality of life, and increasing the risk of institutional admission. For example, there have been some cases where people with ID have been resettled in the community and showed a worsening of their mental or behavioral disorder (Nottestad & Linaker, 1999). Some people were also found to increase their use of local health and mental health services (Kon & Bouras, 1997).

A research project, funded by the BIOMED II Programme of the European Community, was conducted in five European countries (Austria, Greece, England, Ireland, and Spain). The aim of this study was to share information and develop best practice guidelines for people with ID and mental disorders. In order to achieve these aims, it was first necessary to evaluate the current provision of mental health and disability services. Data was collected from each country through in-depth interviews with key service providers and government officials as well as through postal questionnaires and review of research literature, policy, and legislation. The project found increased prevalence of mental disorders, inadequate generic service provision, a need for specialist mental_health services, improved interconnections of services, and development of training—particularly for first-level care workers in community day and residential facilities. It also found that policies on how to provide these services were unclear, especially at a legislative level (Holt et al., 2000). Policy and legislation in these European countries tends to separate the disability aspects of people with ID from their mental disorders. This is also true in most states in the U.S. Consequently, the service needs of this group remain largely invisible. This might be a direct reflection of a lack of policy clarity and legislation, or it could be due to a failure to implement existing guidelines. The effect on the lives of people with ID, their families, and their caregivers has been detrimental. They are frequently bounced back and forth between systems (mental health and ID) without receiving the services that they need. At times, there is a significant delay before they are connected with any service whatsoever.

On the other hand, the last decade has seen the development of more individualized, empowering, and inclusive approaches to services for people with ID. Most of these developments are based on a process of person-centered planning, which is defined in the recently published British Government's white paper, "Valuing People," as "a mechanism for reflecting the needs and preferences of a person with ID and covers issues such as housing, education, employment, and leisure" (Department of Health, 2001, p. 49). It means that planning should start with the individual rather than the services, and planning should take into account the individuals' wishes.

BEHAVIOR DISTURBANCES AND MENTAL DISORDERS

Behavior disturbances are the most common reason for which people with ID are referred for psychiatric assessment (Day, 1985; Jacobson, 1998). However, having a formal diagnosis of a mental disorder rather than a non-specific description of a "behavior disorder" is important, because it may lead to a specific treatment. It may also be of prognostic significance, as there is a body of literature describing the likely effects of treatment for any given disorder. It is also necessary for planning appropriate services, and ensuring that during research the studies look at the most homogeneous group of people possible.

There has been considerable uncertainty regarding the relationship between behavior disturbances and mental disorders that, in many cases, overlap. Understanding the possible links between the two is important, from a theoretical and a clinical perspective, as greater understanding may lead to the subsequent development of more effective treatment methods (Emerson, Moss, & Kiernan, 1999). It is possible that mental disorders underlie or exacerbate behavior disturbances. For example, some forms of self-injurious behavior may be associated with obsessive-compulsive disorder and others with fluctuations of mood states with affective disorders. (See Chapter 5.)

SERVICE MODELS

In line with the principles of normalization, social inclusion, and the human rights movement, there has been a tendency to believe that mental disorders in people with ID could be adequately served within mainstream mental health services. However, services are needed from both the ID network and the mental health system and should be provided in an integrated way, preferably by those who have an understanding of both systems. This allows for more appropriate treatment and support.

Community-Based, Non-Institutional Service Model

The emphasis on community-based, non-institutional services has meant that deficiencies in the provision of care are much more obvious. Individuals are no longer hidden away in institutions but now move about within the community. They must also receive all of their services including mental health care from community providers. Community services do not have the same structures to provide "safety" to others or to contain problems such as aggression or suicide attempts, as the institutions or hospitals have, nor do they mask poor quality of care. The prevailing view is that people with ID and mental disorders have often been under-served or inappropriately treated because of inter-organizational barriers. In the U.S. and other countries, where there has been an overall lack of specialist mental health services for people with ID, there are considerable adverse consequences. These include unnecessary hospitalization and lengthy delays in community placements (Davidson, Morris, & Cain, 1999; Jacobson, 1998).

Attempts to provide mainstream mental health services for people with ID have generally proved less than successful because:

- Staff do not have the necessary skills and resources to assess and manage the care of people with ID;
- People with ID may not interact well with people without ID, if admitted to a generic inpatient unit;

- Clients with ID are vulnerable and generally disadvantaged in such settings;
- The pace of ward life may be too fast for them, and it is difficult to gear therapeutic interventions to meet their special needs.

Specialist Services

The need for specialist interdisciplinary, community-based, accessible services for people with ID and mental disorders or behavior disturbances has been increasingly recognized (Bouras & Szymanski, 1997). In the U.K., specialist mental health teams already exist for a number of specialist groups, such as mothers and babies, eating disorders, and ID.

One example of such a team is the specialist mental health in ID service that operates in South East London, England. It has the same characteristics as other specialist teams: a clear definition of the target client group (based, for example, on diagnosis, age, or gender); an explicit range of treatments, a fixed capacity, and well-clarified roles and responsibilities with high levels of training and skill (Burns, 2001). This particular service operates as both a secondary and tertiary service, accepting referrals from PCPs or generic community mental health teams.

The mental health specialist in ID services works closely with both local generic mental health services and local specialist ID health and social care services. It provides outpatient clinics, outreach work, inpatient assessment and treatment, and consultation with community agencies for people with an ID and a mental disorder. It also provides training to care providers.

The clinical team consists of psychiatrists and community psychiatric nurses. Regular input is also received from clinical psychologists, challenging-needs practitioners (specializing mainly in behavior analysis), occupational therapists, speech therapists, and social workers.

The three phases in the provision of clinical services are: assessment, intervention, and follow-up. A structured assessment is carried out by the team using the Assessment and Information Rating Profile (Bouras & Drummond, 1992).

Therapeutic interventions are based on multidisciplinary work, including medication and environmental manipulation as well as psychological treatments such as cognitive behavior therapy. Crisis prevention plans are developed to help families and service providers identify early signs of breakdown and to take appropriate action. Weekly team meetings are held to review progress.

Training is offered to families and caregivers at this stage to help them better understand and respond to the mental health needs of people with ID. This may take the form of seminars, books, or videos as well as modeling and role-playing exercises. Ongoing support and consultation is also provided.

Follow-up is made available for as long as required. Once a patient appears stable, and the agreed upon strategy seems effective, the team maintains quarterly or six-month contact.

Specialized services such as this are required because:
- The diagnosis of mental disorders in people with ID is complex and requires special skills and expertise;
- Highly specialized assessment and treatment techniques are needed for the management of many mental disorders;

- Therapeutic interventions used with the non-ID population often require modification to take into account intellectual, physical, and other emotional limitations;
- Special regimens and careful monitoring of drug treatment is necessary because of the high frequency of side effects and unusual responses;
- Treatment, rehabilitation, and aftercare must take into account any coexisting physical disabilities, which frequently complicate ID, and
- Specialist services maximize staff skills and competencies, increase the probability of effective and successful treatment, and provide a base for teaching, training, and research.

Davidson and colleagues (1999) in a study of service models in America, Canada, England, and Australia found conceptual and operational problems between mental health and ID service systems, and that communication between and access to services was poor. Disputes between the two service systems, as to which is responsible for providing services, can leave people with ID stranded without the appropriate treatment.

Although the need for specialist services has been recognized, in some areas general mental health and ID services continue to be all that is available. In this case:

- Key staff, including medical and nursing staff, should receive appropriate specialist training from ID staff, if working in a mental health service, and mental health staff, if working in an ID service;
- Guidelines on general approaches and management should be drawn up for all staff—both within their own service and jointly with the ID or mental health service, and
- Initiatives should begin to establish, at the minimum, a specialist community team and a specialist inpatient assessment and treatment unit with staff from both systems or staff that have received training from both systems.

BOX 10.1

The Main Elements of a Specialist Mental Health Service

A comprehensive service should provide:
- For all clinical and diagnostic groups including offenders;
- For all age groups including children, adolescents, and the elderly;
- For all levels of ID from borderline to profound;
- Interdisciplinary assessment and interventions by clinical psychologists, psychiatrists, nurses, social workers, and all other relevant disciplines (including teachers);
- A range of services including community outpatient services for diagnosis and treatment, inpatient facilities for acute treatment as well as continuing care, rehabilitation, and aftercare;
- A full range of treatment approaches including drug therapy, behavior therapy, counseling, and psychotherapy;
- Access to mainstream mental health services, when appropriate;
- Organizational and administrative links with both mainstream mental health and ID services;
- Resources to meet residential, recreational, and vocational needs of those with enduring impairments, and
- A high level of awareness of mental health issues by direct support staff.

Whichever model of service provision exists for people with ID and mental disorders, it is vital to monitor the effectiveness of services in order to develop a good evidence base to support both policy and practice.

TREATMENT ISSUES

The issues that are important in the care of people with mental disorders, who do not have an ID, are equally as important in those who do. These issues include minimizing the social, psychological, and biological risk factors that make people more vulnerable to developing a mental disorder or lead to relapse. To the extent possible, it is important to make evidence-based decisions about the use of specific interventions. The following issues are of heightened or unique importance when treating those with both an ID and a mental disorder.

Informed Consent

It is important to consider the wishes and needs of a person with an ID and a mental disorder who is seeking treatment. If possible, such an individual should give informed consent to any intervention. (See Chapter 11 for more details.) A simple explanation of the intervention should be given so that the person understands what it entails, its potential benefits and drawbacks, and any alternatives available. The individual should also understand what is likely to happen if he or she does not have the treatment. This should not pose too many difficulties when working with people with borderline to mild ID and reasonable communication skills. The use of simple language and visual prompts will make it possible to elicit a person's wishes. However, for people with more profound disabilities it may not be possible to get informed consent. The views of those who know the individual well, perhaps either a caregiver, relative, or advocate, can ensure that interventions are made in the person's best interests. The legal framework and accepted practices will vary from state to state.

Sometimes a person may not be capable of giving informed consent because of a mental disorder. If the person is believed to be a significant risk to himself or others, for example, from physical harm or neglect, involuntary treatment may need to be considered. All states have a legal framework from which to address these issues. See Chapter 11 for an extended discussion of informed consent as well as other ethical and legal issues.

The Relative and Caregivers Role

Many interventions rely on the input of relatives and caregivers that are more involved than the mental health care providers in the lives of those with an ID. They must feel confident in the planned intervention for it to be successful, particularly as most treatment takes place in community settings. They too will need careful explanation of the treatment options, providing that the person with ID does not object to their involvement. As with any client, the right of the individual to confidentiality must be respected. It may be that the client wants certain information to be private, but that other matters can be shared. The support of relatives and caregivers is invaluable to the success of any care plan.

Sometimes relatives and partners may be directly involved in treatment, for instance, if family therapy or marital therapy is suggested. They may also benefit from therapy themselves, for instance, counseling or attendance at a self-help or support group to help them cope with the stresses of being caregivers.

Interdisciplinary Team Responsibilities

In the care of someone with ID and a mental disorder, there may well be professionals from many different services involved, along with the client and family or caregivers. It is important that someone has the primary responsibility for coordinating this input and monitoring the person's progress. A plan must be established that includes review dates, methods of monitoring, and what to do in case of any problems or setbacks. The entire team must be aware of early signs of relapse as well as how to respond to this and any perceived risks to the individual or others. All of this information should be incorporated into a written document for all involved. This document should include an accessible version that uses simple language making it easy to understand for the person with a mental disorder.

SERVICE INTERFACES

Though people with ID should be enabled to access general mental health services whenever possible, these services often do not meet the needs of this group of people either in community settings or in hospitals. This reflects a number of issues including staff training (community mental health centers feel that they do not have the necessary skills), resources (pressure on services so that people with ID can be viewed as taking scarce resources from individuals without ID), and the vulnerability of those with ID (general psychiatric environments can be volatile and potentially violent).

Protocols for collaboration between ID services, specialist mental health services for

Figure 10.1
Organizational Interfaces of Mental Health and ID Services for People with ID and MD

ID Services

Habilitation Model

Skills Development
Needs Assessment
- Day Treatment Programs
- Day Habilitation
- Work Training & Sheltered Work
- Residential Programs
- Institutions
- Group Homes
- Supported Independent Living
- Residential Habilitation

Specialist MH Service for People with ID & MD's

MH Services

Recovery Model

Psychiatric Evaluation
Psychotherapies
- Outpatient Treatment
- Day Treatment
- Individual & Group Therapies
- Inpatient Treatment
- Long-term Facilities
- Mental Illness Chemical Dependence
- Acute Units in General Hospitals
- Acute Units in Academic Centers

people with ID, and mainstream mental health services are very useful. The organizational and funding implications of achieving this also need to be agreed upon.

If alternatives to inpatient treatment are to be sought, whenever possible, for people with ID and mental disorders, the skills of individuals supporting them in their home, whether family members or paid caregivers, will need to be increased. At present, many such caregivers have no expertise in the care of people with an ID and a mental disorder. This is reflected in the difficulty of discharging people with ID and mental disorders from general psychiatric in-patient units to suitable community placements.

For specialist services to be able to work with people in the community, the knowledge base of direct caregivers will need to be improved. Caregivers must feel confident in carrying through and monitoring interventions in collaboration with specialist services. Figure 10.1 depicts a schematic drawing of an idealized organizational structure for an integrated service system for individuals with ID and mental disorders.

Inpatient Facilities

There should be a sufficient number of treatment sites for individuals with ID to provide separate settings for people with mental disorders, people with behavior disturbances, and offenders—with specialized treatment programs developed for each group. Mixing these groups in a single multipurpose unit makes it difficult to develop specific treatment programs. Specialist services, including residential treatment units with appropriate levels of security, are required for offenders with ID.

Community Facilities

The complexity and chronicity of many mental disorders suffered by people with ID often precludes their immediate return to ordinary community facilities. Such individuals require specialized community settings with a structured environment and specially trained staff. While some will only need these services short-term, others will need them long-term. Fletcher and colleagues (1999) recognize that no one model of community care will suit all. As such, a full range of alternatives should be available to enhance an individual's capacity for community living. The individual receiving residential services should be allowed to have as much comfort, ownership, and autonomy as possible.

Specialized community services for rehabilitation and aftercare include:
- Support personnel and specialist teams;
- Day treatment facilities;
- Training and recreational facilities, and
- Community residences.

Need for a Conceptual Framework of Services

Moss and colleagues (2000) postulated a Matrix Model to guide the development and evaluation of services for people with ID and mental disorders. The Matrix Model has two dimensions: a geographical one, which refers to the level of focus (national, state and consumer/client), and a temporal one, which refers to three phases (input, processes, and outcomes). Using these two dimensions, a matrix is constructed that focuses on critical issues for

Figure 10.2
Matrix Model for People with ID & MDs

Level of Focus	Temporal Dimension		
	Inputs	Processes	Outcomes
National	National laws or policies affecting expenditure and national standards of mental health care for people with ID	Identifying at risk and under-served segments of the population	Identifying existing shortcomings in services
State	Existing local services for people with ID	Identifying cases, monitoring referral patterns, treatments, and costs	Improved case identification, improved cost-effectiveness
Customer/Client	Knowledge about treatments and their effectiveness in people with ID	Assessment, treatment, and monitoring of individual cases	Improved outcomes in terms of symptoms, patients quality of life, etc.

community mental health services for people with ID and mental disorders. Figure 10.2 shows the matrix and examples of the kind of information that could be inserted.

This model can facilitate the understanding of how services operate by explaining clinical events in terms of their location in time and space. This is the "where" and "when" that helps with understanding the "how" and "why". Two major advantages can be seen for the adoption of such a model. First, it provides a logical framework for identifying areas for research and development. Secondly, it offers a way of identifying common service dimensions, offering the possibility of comparing and evaluating services operating in diverse national contexts. These factors are particularly relevant to mental health services for people with ID, which are characterized by the involvement of a variety of agencies and organizations, strong ideologies, and conflicting professional views.

The Matrix Model can also be used to prioritize actions that will assist clinicians, planners, administrators, managers, commissioners of services, and clients and their caregivers to develop local-service responses. The actions necessary in each area will be specific to local circumstances. One of the issues likely to require action in many areas is to ensure that quality standards, equivalent to those used for physical health care services, are applied to mental health services, including for those with ID. The Matrix Model could be used to assist in the assessment of local community and clients' needs. It could also be used to develop a research agenda for people with ID and mental disorders to improve diagnosis and detection of mental disorders in this population, to identify their causes, and to evaluate treatment outcomes.

SUMMARY

Despite the development of person-centered planning, the mental health needs of those with ID and mental disorders continue to be overlooked and remain grossly unmet. More efforts are required from all concerned to address this major gap constructively and in a manner of evidence-based practice.

The needs of people with ID and mental disorders are complex; they involve interconnected clinical, organizational, and service factors. Achieving sustainable improvements in mental health service provision will need coherent policies to guide its development. For instance, the agencies responsible for regulating such services should seek evidence that service providers are taking appropriate steps to meet the mental health needs of this population. Broadly speaking, there needs to be a commitment to an evidence-based approach, with treatment and interventions for this population selected and used on the basis of research evidence of their efficacy and clinical evidence of effectiveness. It must be recognized that all levels of staff have a contribution to make in the assessment process, the provision of treatment, and the longer-term support of the individual and his or her caregivers. At present, existing services have reached a crisis point characterized by unclear policies, inter-agency disagreements and limited service responses. This situation presents unpredictable consequences for the quality of life of people with ID and mental disorders, their families, and their caregivers.

REFERENCES

Allen, D. & Felce, D. (1999). Service responses to challenging behavior in psychiatric and behavioural disorders. In N. Bouras (Ed.). *Developmental disabilities and intellectual disabilities* (pp. 279-294). Cambridge University Press.

Bouras, N. & Drummond, C. (1992) Behaviour and psychiatric disorders of people with mental handicaps, living in the community. *Journal of Intellectual Disability Research, 36*, 349-357.

Bouras, N. & Szymanski, L. (1997). Services for people with intellectual disabilities and mental disorders: U.S. - U.K. Comparative Overview. *International Journal of Social Psychiatry, 43*, 64-71.

Burns, T. (2001). Generic versus specialist mental health teams. In G. Thornicroft & G. Szmukler (Eds.) *Textbook of community psychiatry* (pp. 231-241). Oxford University Press.

Davidson, P. W., Morris, D., & Cain, N, N. (1999). Community services for people with psychiatric disorders and ID and psychiatric or severe behavior disorders. In N. Bouras (Ed.). *Disabilities psychiatric and behavioural disorders in developmental disabilities and intellectual* (pp 359-372). Cambridge University Press.

Day, K. (1985). Psychiatric disorder in the middle-aged and elderly mentally handicapped. *British Journal of Psychiatry, 147*, 660-667.

Deb, S., Matthews, T., Holt, G., & Bouras, N. (2001). Practice guidelines for assessment and diagnosis of mental health problems. *Adults with Intellectual Disability.* Brighton, England: Pavilion Publishing.

Department of Health (2001). *Valuing people: A new strategy for learning disability for the 21st century.* London: HMSO.

Dosen, A. (1993). Diagnosis and treatment of psychiatric and behavioural disorders in mentally retarded individuals: The state of the art. *Journal of Intellectual Disability Research, 37*, Supplement I, 1-7.

Emerson, E. & Hatton, C. (1995). *Moving Out: Relocation from Hospital to Community.* London: HMSO.

Emerson, E., Moss, S., & Kiernan, C. (1999). The relationship between challenging behavior and psychiatric disorders in people with severe intellectual disabilities. In N. Bouras (Ed.), *Psychiatric and behavioural disorders in intellectual disabilities.* Cambridge University Press.

Fletcher, R. J., Beasley, J. and Jacobson, J. W. (1999). Support service systems for people with dual diagnosis in the U.S. In N. Bouras, (Ed.), *Psychiatric and behavioural disorders in developmental disabilities and intellectual disabilities* (pp. 373-390). Cambridge University Press.

Gardner, W. I., Graeber, J. I., & Cole, C. L. (1996). Behavior therapies: A multimodal diagnostic and intervention model. In J. W. Jacobson & J. A. Mulick (Eds.), *Manual of diagnosis and professional practice in Intellectual Disabilities* (pp. 355-370). Washington, DC: American Psychological Association.

Gardner, W. I. & Whalen, J. P. (1996). Discussion: A multimodal behavior analytic model for evaluating the effects of medical problems on nonspecific behavioral symptoms in persons with developmental disabilities. *Behavioral Interventions, 11,* 147-163.

Hatton, C., Emerson, E., & Kiernan, C. (1995). People in institutions in Europe. *Intellectual Disabilities, 33*, 132.

Holt, G., Costello, H., Bouras, N., Diareme, S., Hillery, H., Moss, S., et al. (2000). BIOMED-MEROPE Project: Service provision for adults with intellectual disabilities: A European comparison. *Journal Intellectual Disability Research, 44*, 685-696.

Jacobson J. (1998). Psychological services utilization: Relationship to severity of behavior problems in intellectual disability services. *Journal of Intellectual Disability Research, 42*, 307-15.

Kon, Y. & Bouras, N. (1997). Psychiatric follow-up and health services utilisation for people with learning disabilities. *The British Journal of Developmental Disabilities, 84*, 20-26.

Moss S., Bouras N., & Holt G. (2000). Mental health services for people with intellectual disabilities: A conceptual framework. *Journal Intellectual Disability Research, 44*, pp 97-107.

Moss, S. C., Prosser, H., Costello, H., Simpson, N., Patel, P., Rowe, S., et al. (1998). Reliability and validity of the PAS-ADD checklist for detecting disorders in adults with intellectual disability, *Journal of Intellectual Disability Research, 42*(2) 173-183.

Nottestad J. A. & Linaker O. M. (1999). Psychiatric health needs and services before and after complete deinstitutionalisation of people with intellectual disabilities. *Journal of Intellectual Disability Research, 43*, 523-530.

11

Ethical and Legal Issues

Christine D. Cea and Celia B. Fisher[1]

INTRODUCTION

It has been recognized in recent years that persons with ID may also have mental health needs. This recognition has increased practitioners' understanding of mental disorders in this population and has brought about new treatment modalities. In turn, these advances have provided adults with ID greater freedom to live and work in the community and to experience a full range of decision-making opportunities. However, the treatment of adults with mental disorders and ID poses complex legal and ethical questions regarding their capacity to give informed, rational, and voluntary consent to interventions designed to test the efficacy of these treatments. In addition, the invasive nature of many treatments (e.g., psychopharmacological medications, behavioral techniques, therapeutic interventions, voluntary hospitalization) raises complex issues for practitioners and family members regarding how to appropriately balance the right of individuals with ID and mental disorders to make treatment decisions with the obligation of practitioners and caretakers to ensure that these decisions are in the client's best interest (Ellis, 1992; Fisher, 1999).

This chapter begins with a discussion of the moral foundation and legal requirements of informed consent, including how they apply to persons with mental disorders and ID, and how characteristics of the disorder may affect indivduals' ability to make informed and voluntary consent decisions. A general framework for assessing consent capacity is presented, along with information about surrogate decision-making and guardianship for persons with mild ID who are unable to make treatment decisions for themselves. The chapter closes with a detailed description of the required information in the disclosure given to clients and prospective research participants prior to obtaining their consent. Methods for increasing disclosure understanding and assessing the voluntary nature of decision-making in this population are also presented.

MORAL FOUNDATIONS OF INFORMED CONSENT

The requirement for informed consent for treatment and research rests on the principle of respect for individual privacy and autonomy. However, when working with populations with questionable capacity to consent, the principles of beneficence and justice also serve to guide the moral action of practitioners and scientists in obtaining informed consent (American Psychological Association Ethical Principles and Codes of Conduct, APA, 2002; National Commission for the Protection of Human Subjects in Biomedical and Behavioral Research, 1979).

Respect for Autonomy

The principle of *respect for autonomy* acknowledges both the human capacity for self-determination and the obligation to protect persons with diminished autonomy. Information required to ensure individuals' rights to self-governance include the nature of treatment and research procedures, potential risks and benefits of participation, the extent and limits of confidentiality, the voluntary nature of participation, and alternative treatments or procedures that are available. The ethical challenge for those working with adults with ID and comorbid mental disorders is to balance the obligation to respect their right to be treated as members of the moral community, with the need to ensure that ill-informed or incompetent decisions will not place their welfare in jeopardy (Ellis, 1992; Fisher, 1999).

Beneficence

The principle of *beneficence* reflects the moral and ethical obligation of practitioners and scientists to maximize benefits to others and minimize potential harm and suffering. How the principle of beneficence is put into practice often depends upon the way that it is modified by the other ethical principles, especially the principle of respect for autonomy. For example, Churchill (1995) suggests that respect for autonomy means that the client or potential research participant defines what he or she considers *good*. Beneficence not defined in the same way may lead to paternalistic decision-making that unnecessarily conflicts with clients' perspectives (Churchill, 1995; Faden & Beauchamp, 1986). The presumption of incompetence for individuals with ID is often so common that both individuals diagnosed with such impairments and those without ID who work with and care for them, often consider diminished autonomy natural and necessary (Ellis, 1992).

Justice

The principle of *justice* signifies the right to share equally in the distribution of treatments and their risks and benefits. Justice is realized when allocation of services are distributed equally and fairly to all members of society (Faden et al., 1986). Unjust practices toward persons with mental disorders were common during the nineteenth and early twentieth centuries, when clients were confined to institutions and denied the benefits of improved medical treatment that were offered to non-institutionalized clients. In a now infamous study conducted at the Willowbrook State School, institutionalized children with ID were used as a sample of convenience to develop a vaccine for infectious hepatitis. Not only were residents and their parents not fully appraised of the risks and voluntary nature of participation, but many children also subsequently contracted the illness (Herr, 1983).

LEGAL REQUIREMENTS OF INFORMED CONSENT

Traditionally, it has been the role of the courts to interpret the ethical principles of autonomy, beneficence, and justice with respect to the legal requirements of informed consent (Faden et al., 1986). These legal requirements were introduced into case law in 1957 as the Doctrine of Informed Consent.

Evolving primarily from court cases in which clients were inadequately informed by physicians prior to treatment (e.g., *Schloendorff v. Society of New York Hospitals*, 1914; *Natanson v. Klein*, 1960), the Doctrine of Informed Consent is intended to safeguard individual rights to self-determination by requiring that the client: (1) be provided sufficient *information* regarding the nature and purpose of the treatment, (2) has the *capacity* to understand treatment information and make a rational choice, and (3) makes a *voluntary* decision to be treated. All three elements of informed consent must be present in order to legally safeguard autonomous decision-making.

Knowledge

The knowledge requirement of informed consent obligates practitioners and clinical researchers to provide clients with sufficient information to make an informed decision about whether they wish to receive treatment or to participate in an experimental investigation of a new treatment. Such information must include a description of risks and potential benefits, discomforts, and side effects of a proposed treatment, available alternatives, and the consequences of no treatment at all. The information must be presented in a way that is understandable to the person. Practitioners must, to the extent possible, adapt disclosure information to the individual's level of comprehension and language ability and be free of technical jargon (Hurley & O'Sullivan, 1999). It is also important that the practitioner seeking consent offers to answer any questions, and that the client is allowed the opportunity to consult with others not directly involved (Turnbull, 1977).

Capacity

The second requirement, capacity, calls for an individual to have the ability to understand and reason about disclosure information to make an informed and voluntary choice. By law, all adults are presumed to have decision-making capacity, unless it is proven otherwise (O'Sullivan, 1999) and a diagnosis of ID cannot be accepted as presumption of decisional incompetence (Bersoff, Glass, & Blain, 1994; Conditions of Participation, 1988; Dinerstein, 1994; Lindsay & Luckasson, 1991; *Reenie v. Klein*, 1982; *Rogers v. Okin*, 1982; Wolfensberger, 1972). The presence of a mental disorder and ID, therefore, is not a *de facto* judgment of consent impairment. To achieve an appropriate balance between client rights and client protection, evaluation of consent capacity for persons with mental disorders and ID must take into consideration the specific characteristics of the individual and the complexity of the decision at hand (Ellis, 1992; Fisher, 1999; 2003).

Voluntariness

The third requirement, voluntariness, is central to the concept of individual autonomy. This element requires that the client's consent is free from coercion, persuasion, manipulation, or undue influence. From an ethical perspective, therefore, regardless of good intentions, failure to allow a person with a mental disorder and ID the right to accept or refuse treatment can violate the moral principle of respect for individual autonomy. From a legal perspective, a client's decision about treatment is not effective if it has not been given voluntarily (Appelbaum, Lidz, & Meisel, 1987). For people with mental disorders and ID, the issue of voluntariness is magnified because deficits in intellectual functioning, lack of experience, and lack of opportunity to make autonomous decisions, compounded by emotional or personality disorders makes them uniquely susceptible to pressure or coercion to accept treatment. Such individuals may also be eager to please and not disappoint or anger staff or family members whose opinions may have strong influence (Fisher, 1999; Hurley & O'Sullivan, 1999) and upon whom they are dependent.

EVALUATING CONSENT CAPACITY

The question of an individual's capacity to consent or refuse medical intervention or to participate in clinical research rests on his or her ability for informed decision-making. Although, having a mental disorder and ID is no longer accepted as a presumption of incompetence, the characteristics and course of the disability and societal limitations placed on individuals diagnosed as such, shape issues of consent in unique ways (Ellis, 1992). Within the group of people classified as having ID, there is variability in functioning, ranging from those who are totally dependent to those who are independent. Moreover, the presence of a mental disorder and its relevant features may affect competent decision-making of those functioning even at the mildest levels of ID. Thus, the potential for impaired decisional capacity of people with ID may suffer further from mental disorders that can be persistent, sporadic, episodic, or cyclical in nature. Given the large percentage of persons with mental disorders and ID, assessment of decision relevant features of an individual's mental disorder is critical to understanding his or her capacity to give informed consent (Freedman, 1998).

STANDARDS FOR DETERMINING CONSENT CAPACITY

At present, there is little agreement on a generally accepted definition of consent capacity, nor are there established standards to guide its determination. State law has traditionally determined the decision regarding an individual's capacity to consent, with courts choosing from a number of standards individually applied on a case-by-case basis and varying from jurisdiction to jurisdiction.

Appelbaum and his colleagues (Appelbaum & Grisso, 1988; Appelbaum & Roth, 1982; Grisso & Appelbaum, 1998) developed the most influential framework for evaluating capacity to consent based on a consideration of judicial standards in which these clinical and legal decisions are made. They propose that the capacity to provide informed consent for treatment or research participation can be evaluated within four increasingly demanding psycho-legal standards of consent capacity. The first and least stringent of these standards is the ability to *communicate a choice* about treatment or research participation. The second standard pertains to the ability to *understand factual information* about the nature of the treatment or research as well as the risks and benefits of the proposals of each. The third standard, *appreciation of the situation and its consequences*, requires that the client or potential research participant understands not only the risks and benefits, but also the cognitive and emotional implications of the treatment or research participation, as they apply to his or her own circumstances. The fourth and final standard, *rational manipulation of information*, is the most cognitively complex and requires the ability to weigh the risks and benefits of the proposed treatment or research, when making a choice, and to arrive at a *reasonable* outcome of choice.

Recently, the American Psychiatric Association (APA, 1998) sited the relevancy of the same four psycho-legal standards in assessing a client's capacity to make treatment and research decisions, suggesting that most states utilize one or more of these standards in determining whether clients and/or research subjects have the capacity to make their own decisions. The APA advises practitioners and research scientists to familiarize themselves with the specific standards that apply in their particular jurisdiction and to consult with legal counsel, if necessary. However, there is little consensus on which of the psycho-legal standards should be applied, leading to concern that adults with ID and mental disorders may be held to a higher standard of decisional competence than individuals with ID without mental disorders (Fisher, 1999).

SURROGATE DECISION-MAKING AND GUARDIANSHIP

At 18 years of age all persons are presumed competent to make their own decisions, unless it is has been legally determined that they are incapable of doing so. There will be instances in which the capacity of adults with mental disorders and ID to make informed, rational, and voluntary consent decisions will be impaired (Freedman, 1998). For many, this capacity will vary with the situation for which consent is sought (Fisher, 2002, 2003). In the case of medical treatment, a person may be able to give consent to treatments that are of low risk and low invasiveness such as routine tests and medical examinations, but not be able to understand or balance the risks and benefits of treatments that are more complicated and present greater probabilities of risk such as surgery or psychotropic medications (Hurley et al., 1999). In such instances, a parent or legal guardian is usually sought to either assist the decision-making or serve as a surrogate.

Surrogate Decision-making for Medical Treatment

Surrogate decision-making laws allow parents or other close family members of persons with diminished capacity to consent to routine medical treatment without involving the courts, if the person who lacks capacity is willing to be treated (Freedman, 1998; Hurley et al., 1999). The surrogate can use *substitute judgment*, defined as making a treatment judgment based upon the surrogate's understanding of what the individual would have decided if he or she were capable of decision-making. When the surrogate may not have direct knowledge of the individual's wishes, the surrogate may make decisions in the *best interests* of the person by weighing the benefits and risks of treatment against the risks of no treatment (Freedman, 1998; O'Sullivan, 1999). In most states, however, a surrogate cannot give consent for treatment if the person in question actively refuses to be treated or for certain treatments such as "forcible medication with antipsychotic drugs, electroconvulsive therapy, sterilization, and abortion" (Hurley et al., 1999, p.49).

Guardianship

Guardianship laws permit parents or another concerned individual (e.g., a sibling) to petition courts in their state to become guardians of adults who have little or no decision-making capacity by granting them legal responsibility to make *best interest* decisions for their adult child (or sibling). Guardianship can be *of the person* or *of property*. Guardianship of the person allows the guardian to be the decision-maker for all daily decisions in the life of the person who is determined incapacitated (e.g., where they live, what treatments they receive, managing their funds). Guardianship of property allows the guardian to handle all of the assets and income on behalf of the individual. In some states, a petition for temporary guardianship may also be sought for the purpose of making time-limited decisions, such as a specific medical procedure for which the individual with ID cannot consent.

As with other issues of decision-making by and for people with mental disorders and ID, decisions about whether it is necessary to seek guardianship of a particular individual and whether or not to accept or refuse treatment for the same person as a surrogate or guardian, brings up the complex issue of how to best weigh the adult's right to autonomy with the obligation to provide protection and advocacy that is in his or her best interest. For a more thorough discussion of guardianship and surrogate decision-making, see *A Guide to Consent* by Dinerstein, Herr, and O'Sullivan (1999).

Suggestions

Informed consent is a process in which the primary responsibility of practitioners and research scientists is to decide whether an individual understands information specific to the treatment or research study and that he or she has the capacity to make a voluntary decision (Fisher, 1999; Hurley et al., 1999). While limited decisional capacity need not prevent decision-making in treatment or research contexts, the ethical dilemma for practitioners, scientists, and family members lies in attempting to achieve a proper balance of risks versus benefits and freedom to choose versus protection from harm.

It is incumbent upon practitioners and clinical scientists to not only understand the influence of the specific features of ID on informed decision-making of people with mental disorders and ID, but to also be sensitive to the potential implication of their mental disorder (e.g., depression, psychosis) on consent capacity. For lower levels of impairment, this understanding can help professionals adjust standard consent methods and procedures to the needs of the client and to implement more protective procedures for higher levels of impairment.

INFORMED CONSENT PROCEDURES

A fundamental requirement of informed consent is that it be *informed*, that is, the client or prospective research participant must be provided with specific information in order to ensure that a valid decision is made. Expert consensus and federal guidelines (AAID, 2000, p.169; DHHS, 1991) suggests that this information include:
- A description of the nature of the problem;
- The specific signs and symptoms that will be the targets of treatment;
- A description of the proposed treatment and who will provide it;
- Any alternative treatments;
- The benefits and risks of the proposed treatment and alternatives;
- The individual's right to refuse treatment or participation, and
- The right to change one's mind and withdraw from the treatment or research at any time without consequences.

The disclosure should also include a statement regarding confidentiality that ensures prospective clients or research participants of their right to privacy of information.

Increasing Disclosure Understanding

Because people with mental disorders and ID may have limited consent capacity, methods to increase understanding of disclosure information must be used in order to ensure that valid and informed decisions are made. It is recommended that disclosure information for treatment or research participation involving adults with ID be free of technical information and use short sentences and concrete language (Cea & Fisher, 2003; Hurley et al., 1999). Careful explanations and repetition of information, teaching materials such as pictures, videotapes, and demonstration models can also enhance consent comprehension. In addition, speaking slowly to allow time for processing and communicating a willingness to answer any and all questions may also enhance consent capacity. Questions should be asked in several ways to ensure that the client or research participant understands the information. For example, *yes* and *no* questions should be kept to a minimum to avoid response bias. If the prospective clients or research participants can express themselves verbally, procedures such as asking for an explanation of the disclosure information in their own words can help evaluate whether they grasp what is being said.

Assessing Voluntariness

While it is assumed that all adults can give voluntary consent, the circumstances of the individual may influence whether or not consent is truly voluntarily given. It is often difficult to determine the amount of real or perceived coercion experienced by vulnerable individuals, such as people with mental disorders and ID (Ellis, 1992). Physical and social restrictions in a client's living environment (e.g., institutional settings, community residences), lack of experience with autonomous decision making, and treatment preferences expressed by staff and family members can make persons with mental disorders and ID more vulnerable to unintentional or subtle forms of coercion or exploitation (Ellis, 1992, Hurley et al., 1999; Turnbull, 1977). Adults with mental disorders and ID may be eager to please and not disappoint staff and family members, or believe it is inappropriate to refuse treatments or research recruitment from authority figures such as doctors and clinical investigators. Furthermore, their freedom to withdraw from the study may be compromised because they may not be able to recognize or report negative side effects of medications, may suffer these in silence, or act out behaviorally until the symptoms are recognized and addressed by others (Hurley et al., 1999).

While it may not be possible to detect every factor that might diminish decision-making in this population, it is possible to reduce the perceived control of people with a mental disorder and ID in treatment and research settings. First, because the environment (examining room, clinic, or other unfamiliar institutional setting) may exert pressure on clients to comply with treatment proposals, the assessment of consent should be conducted in a less threatening context (e.g., office versus examining room) or in settings familiar to the individual. If possible, the consent should be obtained by someone that the client knows and trusts and in the presence of a trusted family member or friend (Freedman, 1998). Finally, with regard to recruitment to participate in studies testing new treatments, inducements for participation may unduly influence decision-making in people with mental disorders and ID. Prior to offering compensation, clinical scientists should consult with clients, residential staff, or family members regarding what level and type of payment would be consistent with the client's everyday opportunities.

SUMMARY

The issue of consent for treatment or research participation of individuals with mental disorders and ID poses complex ethical challenges for families, health care practitioners, and researchers in trying to balance respect for client autonomy with the obligation to protect client welfare. Each person with a mental disorder and ID is unique. Individual capacities need to be considered, and the implications of these capacities to informed decision-making clearly understood. Once it is determined that a person with mental disorders and ID is unable to make decisions for him or herself, these decisions can be made by an informed surrogate decision-maker or guardian whose decisions reflect the client's preferences and concerns.

REFERENCES

American Association on Intellectual Disabilities (2000). Informed consent. Expert Consensus Guideline Series: Treatment of Psychiatric and Behavioral Problems in Intellectual Disabilities.

American Psychiatric Association (1998). Guidelines for assessing the decision-making capacities of potential research subjects with cognitive impairments. *American Journal of Psychiatry, 155*(11), 1649-1650.

American Psychological Association (2002). Ethical principles of psychologists and code of conduct. *American Psychologist, 57*.

Appelbaum, P. S. & Grisso, T. (1988). Assessing clients' capacities to consent to treatment. *New England Journal of Medicine, 319* (25), 1635-1638.

Appelbaum, P. S. & Roth, L. H. (1982). Competency to consent to research: A psychiatric overview. *Archives of General Psychiatry, 39*, 951-958.

Appelbaum, P. S., Lidz, C. W., & Meisel, A. (1987). *Informed consent: Legal theory and clinical practice.* New York: Oxford University Press.

Bersoff, D. N., Glass, D. J., & Blain, N. (1994). Legal issues in the assessment and treatment of individuals with dual diagnoses. *Journal of Consulting and Clinical Psychology, 62*, 55-62.

Cea, D. C., & Fisher, C. B. (2003). Health care decision-making by adults with mental retardation. *Mental Retardation, 41*, 78-87.

Churchill, L. R. (1995). Beneficence. In W. T. Reich (Ed.), *Encyclopedia of bioethics* (Volume 1, pp. 243-247). New York: Simon, Schuster & MacMillan.

Conditions of Participation for Intermediate Care Facilities for the Mentally Retarded, 42 CFR Subchapter E Part 483. (1988). Federal Register, 53(107), 20448-20505.

Dinerstein, R. D. (1994). Revising the consent handbook: From consent to choice. *AAMR News and Notes, 7*, 1.

Dinerstein, R. D., Herr, S. S., & O'Sullivan, J. L. (Eds.). (1999). *A guide to consent.* Washington, DC: American Association on Intellectual Disabilities.

Department of Health and Human Services [DHHS] (1991, August). Title 45 Public Welfare, Part 46, Code of Federal Regulations, Protection of Human Subjects.

Ellis, J. W. (1992). Decisions by and for people with intellectual disabilities: Balancing considerations of autonomy and protection. *Villanova Law Review, 37*, 1799-1809.

Faden, R. R. & Beauchamp, T. L. (1986). *A history and theory of informed consent.* New York: Oxford University Press.

Fisher, C. B., (1999). Relational ethics and research with vulnerable populations. Reports on research involving persons with Mental Disorders that may affect decision-making capacity Vol. II, (pp. 29-49). Commissioned papers by the National Bioethics Advisory Commission. Rockville, MD.

Fisher, C. B. (2002). A goodness-of-fit ethic of informed consent. *Urban Law Journal, 30,* 159-171.

Fisher, C. B. (2003). A goodness-of-fit ethic for informed consent to research involving persons with Intellectual Disabilities and developmental disabilities. *Mental Retardation and Developmental Disabilities Research Reviews 9,* 27-31.

Freedman, R. I. (1998). Use of advance directives: Facilitating health care decisions by adults with Intellectual Disabilities and their families. *Intellectual Disabilities, 36*(6), 444-456.

Grisso, T. & Appelbaum, P. S. (1998). Assessing competence to consent to treatment. New York: Oxford University Press.

Herr, S. S. (1983). *Rights and advocacy for retarded people.* Lexington, MA: D. C. Heath & Company.

Hurley, A. D. & O'Sullivan, J. L. (1999). Informed Consent for Health Care. In R. D. Dinerstein, S. S. Herr, & J. L. O'Sullivan (Eds.). *A guide to consent.* Washington, DC: American Association on Intellectual Disabilities.

Lindsay, P. & Luckasson, R. (1991). Consent screening interview for community residential placement: Report on the initial pilot study data. *Intellectual Disabilities, 20,* 119-124. *Natanson v. Kline, 350 P.2d 1093 (1960).*

National Commission for the Practice of Human Subjects in Biomedical and Behavioral Research (1979). The Belmont Report: Ethical principles and guidelines for the protection of human subjects of research (GPO 887-809). Washington, DC: U.S. Government Printing Office.

O'Sullivan, J. L. (1999). Adult Guardianship and Alternatives. In R. D. Dinerstein, S. S. Herr, & J. L. O'Sullivan (Eds.). *A guide to consent.* Washington, DC: American Association on Intellectual Disabilities.

Reenie v. Klein, 462 F. Supp. 1131 (1978); modified, 476 F. Supp. 1294 (1979); 481 F. Supp. 552 (179); modified and remanded, 653 F.2nd 836 (1981); vacated and remanded, 50 YSLW 3998.27 (1982).

Rogers v. Okin, 478 F. Supp. 1342 (1979); affirmed in part, reversed in part, vacated in part, and remanded 643 f.2nd 650 (1980); vacated and remanded sub.nom *Mills v. Rogers* 457 U. W. 291 (1982); certified questions answered sub.nom. *Rogers v. Commissioner of Mental Health*, 390. Mass. 489 (1982).

Schloendorff v. Society of New York Hospitals, 211 N.Y. 125, 126, 105 N.E., 92, 93 (1914).

Turnbull, H. R. (1977). Consent Handbook. Washington, DC: American Association on Mental Deficiency.

Wolfensberger, W. (1972). *The principle of normalization.* Toronto, Canada: National Institute of Intellectual Disabilities.

FOOTNOTE

1. The writing of this chapter was supported by the National Institute of Child Health and Human Development grant #HD39332-02 awarded to C. B. Fisher.

Contributors

JoAnne T. Baxter, C.S.W.
Instructor and Trainer, M.R.D.D. Psychiatric Disorders Clinic
University of Rochester

Nick Bouras, M.D., Ph.D., F.R.C. Psych.
Professor of Psychiatry
Division of Psychological Medicine and Health Service Research Department
Institute of Psychiatry, King's College, London
Estia Centre, Guy's Hospital

Nancy N. Cain, M.D., D.F.A.P.A.
Associate Assistant Professor of Psychiatry
Director of Programs for Mental Disorders and Mental Retardation
University of Rochester School of Medicine and Dentistry

Christine D. Cea, Ph.D.
Marie Doty University Chair in Psychology and
Director, Center for Ethics Education
Fordham University

Amy Cowley, B.Sc. (Hons.)
Guy's-King's St. Thomas's Medical School, York Clinic
Estia Centre, Guy's Hospital

Philip W. Davidson, Ph.D.
Professor of Pediatrics
Director, Strong Center for Developmental Disabilities
University of Rochester School of Medicine and Dentistry

Howard B. Demb, M.D.
Albert Einstein College of Medicine of Yeshiva University

Celia B. Fisher, Ph.D.
Professor of Psychology
Fordham University Center for Ethics Education

Geraldine Holt, M.B.B.S., B.Sc., F.R.C.Psych.
Senior Lecturer in Psychiatry of Learning Disability
Division of Psychological Medicine and Health Service Research Department
Institute of Psychiatry King's College, London
Estia Centre, Guy's Hospital

John W. Jacobson, Ph.D., B.C.B.A.
Instructor
Sage Colleges Center for Behavior Analysis
New York State Office of Intellectual Disabilities and Developmental Disabilities

Jennifer Katz, Ph.D.
Visiting Assistant Professor
Department of Psychology
State University of New York College at Geneseo

Ronald Lee, M.A.
Queens College and Graduate Center
City University of New York

Caroline I. Magyar, Ph.D.
Assistant Professor of Pediatrics
Director, Autism Spectrum Disorders Program
Strong Center for Developmental Disabilities
University of Rochester School of Medicine and Dentistry

John C. Pomeroy, M.B.B.S., M.R.C. Psych.
Associate Professor of Pediatrics and Psychiatry
Director of the Cody Center for Autism and Developmental Disabilities
State University of New York at Stony Brook

Howie Reyer, M.A.
Queens College and Graduate Center
City University of New York

Adrienne Robek, M.A.
Queens College and Graduate Center
City University of New York

Tristram H. Smith, Ph.D.
Assistant Professor of Pediatrics (Psychology)
University of Rochester School of Medicine and Dentistry

Peter Sturmey, Ph.D.
Queens College and Graduate Center
City University of New York

Anthony Villani, M.D.
Rochester Psychiatric Center

About the Editors

Nancy N. Cain, M.D., D.F.A.P.A. has worked in the field of dual diagnosis for many years. As Director of Psychiatric Services for individuals with intellectual disabilities at the University of Rochester Medical Center, she developed a model for providing comprehensive psychiatric care for individuals with ID living in the community. In this settin, Dr. Cain was active in teaching medical students, residents and other health care providers. She has authored publications with a number of colleagues, presented at national and international meetings and done clinical research on aggression, crisis intervention and bipolar disorder in individuals with ID.

Geraldine Holt, M.B.B.S., B.Sc., F.R.C. Psych. is a consultant psychiatrist in Learning Disabilities at South London and the Maudsley NHS Trust and Honorary Senior Lecturer at the Institute of Psychiatry, London. She is a fellow of the Royal College of Psychiatrists, a member of several National and International Associations and has published extensively, including training packages and material.

Philip W. Davidson, Ph.D. is Professor of Pediatrics and Psychiatry at the University of Rochester School of Medicine and Dentistry and the Director of the Strong Center for Developmental Disabilities. He has over one hundred peer-reviewed publications, sixty book chapters and is the editor or co-editor of three books. He serves on the editorial boards of several peer-reviewed journals.

Nick Bouras, M.D., Ph.D., F.R.C. Psych. is Professor of Psychiatry at the Institute of Psychiatry at King's College, London and Consultant Psychiatrist at South London and the Maudsley NHS Trust. He has long experience in mental health and services for people with developmental disabilities. He has published extensively and has edited several books.